Newnham

THE 4 PILLARS OF HEALTH

Your health and well-being made simple!

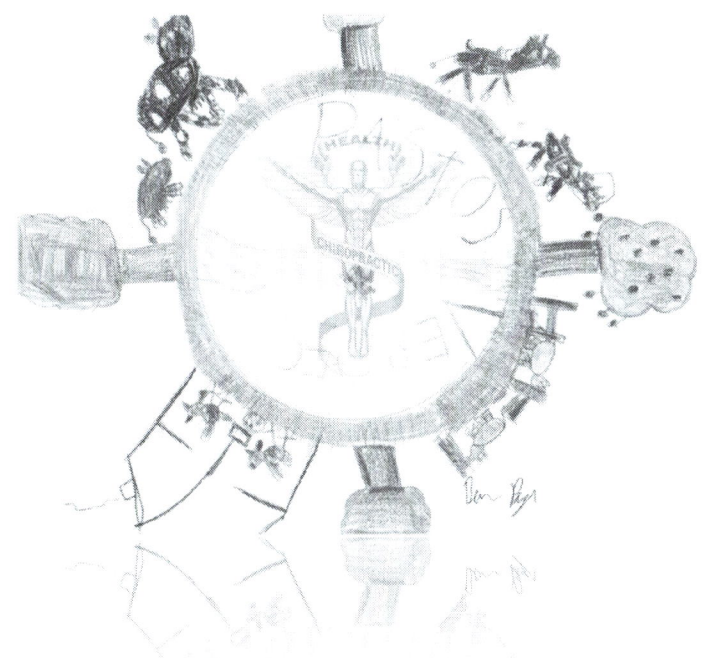

Benjamin David Page, D.C.

3rd edition, 2017 *www.pastosverdesfarm.com*

1

The best monographs are not those that contain only information, but those that convey readers a philosophy, a set of integrated ideas on how to improve one's life. The book of Dr. Page falls amongst those that leave a philosophical imprint on readers, transmit practical knowledge, and at the same time, awaken the curiosity to learn more about the subject.

While most books on preventive or therapeutic medicine tend to adopt radical positions in one way or another (for example, "do not consume animal proteins"), Dr. Page's book shows an uncommonly realistic balance with solid scientific basis. It is the first time I read in a book about health, not only a description of how animals are treated in industrial farms, but also how to raise animals (in this case, free-range chickens) in a healthy, natural way.

The philosophy of individual responsibility that the book transmits is coming from afar. The author is a descendant of chiropractors. His grandfather was already a practitioner, and the book tells us how his desire to heal and help other people has been transmitted from generation to generation within the family.

The book provides practical advice gathered first-hand. When the author is describing how to organize a farm, he explains in detail the importance of dividing the area of cultivation into five zones, planting herbs and vegetables near the house because those plants require frequent attention. It is obvious that the author has managed a farm itself, and that he knows what he is talking about.

The ideas presented in the book are rooted in a spirit of personal independence and self-sufficiency in the maintenance of one's health and well-being. It is a spirit that the author developed in his student days, and that he is now conveying convincingly, giving hands-on advice.

When Dr. Page is writing that, in his daily life, he tries to go on foot whenever he can instead of using his car or public transportation, he is preaching with example. The same thing happens when he is telling us about his morning routine that includes a period of meditation, and drinking a herbal infusion. These are examples that every reader can immediately follow.

Another part of the book that is also providing immediately applicable advice is the chapter on sleep, and on the impact that daily rest has on one's health. Chiropractors are specialists in the nervous system, and they know how to handle psycho-somatic conditions. They know precisely what we have to do in order to improve our sleeping habits.

The book chapters that are dealing with a bad bodily posture (a sign of incipient or present disease) and a bad spiritual posture (what we say to ourselves when we are incorrectly interpreting reality) are providing readers with the necessary guidelines to address those problems, although making it clear that, in severe cases, the help of a specialist is necessary.

While the book begins by graphically describing the life of a sick person (tired, overwhelmed, disoriented), it ends up in an optimistic tone by talking about positive stress (eustress), and how it differs from detrimental stress. Dr. Page is emphasizing the importance of a positive internal dialogue as a basis for a healthy, happy and balanced life. A very interesting book for anyone who wants to take a step forward in his health and well-being.

review written by John Vespasian on March 26, 2018

I would like to thank my wife for all that she does, this would not have happened without her help and support. THANK YOU!!! I have a great wife and two great kids that help me grow so much everyday.

I would like to thank my mom and dad for all the help they have provided in this very long process. THANKS!!!

A special thanks to "Lita" my grandma who helped with financing the edit of this book. I couldn't have done it without you! MUCHAS GRACIAS LITA!!

I would like to send out a thank you to Andrés Ravello, Ray Holt and my mom, Silvia Page, for taking the time to read through the book beforehand. Thanks!!

I would also like to thank all the listeners of my podcasts "The wellness farmer podcast" and en español "El podcast la salud integral"

Health and well-being...9
Finding the desire!..11
The first step in the journey to true health and well-being........11
Who we truly are!...15
Nutrient dense food...19
Gut health and its importance 19
- Meat – one of the important components of our diet.................20
- Vegetables and fruits – important components of our diet...........25
- Fats and oils – not to be scared of. Our bodies need them!........27
- Grains – the one food source we should be eating less of! 34
- The answer to the modern food system!.............................39
- Permaculture – grow food and build soil at the same time!.........42
- Where do I find food that is nutrient dense? 47

Chiropractic Care 53
The forgotten pillar...53
- The First T – Toxins...58
- The Second T – Thoughts..62
- The Third T – Traumas..63
- The stress response – why chiropractic is one of the four pillars to true health..65
- Eustress—the other side of stress..................................71

Natural internal dialogue..79
Exactly that – natural!..79
- The morning routine – a great start!...............................84
- Modern survivalism and the wellness lifestyle......................87

Movement 97
Not just for athletes!...97
- Sleep - movement's companion......................................103
- Posture – the other side of the coin..............................111

Why We Must Get the Word Out! 119

Health and well-being

Health has been made too complex! That is why I am writing this book. I want to help you understand four basic concepts of health – that is it! If you live a lifestyle which involves these four basic concepts holistically, you will find true health and well-being. While health is simple, putting these four concepts into practice is not as easy. But all good things come with work, and the best part about this work is that it is fun and satisfying. To find true health we first have to have a plan that shows us how to find it. That plan is right here, in this book! With a plan, we can reach our destination. Without it, we are lost.

Most people feel lost about what health and wellness really is. There is so much information out there, making it very difficult to know what to do. This is one of the problems – we are bombarded with propaganda daily, and we often don't have time to study things out. If you are reading this, I know you want to find true health and well-being and that you are also willing to make changes in your lifestyle so you can actually feel what it is to be truly healthy. As a chiropractor who has studied extensively about what brings about true health and well-being, and who works personally with many patients, I can say that one of the best feelings I get is seeing my family and patients healthy and well. Let me do the same for you.

What are the 4 pillars of health?

The four pillars are simple concepts however will take work and practice to implement in our lives.

They are:

1. Nutrient dense food grown on fertile soil without chemicals

2. Chiropractic care

3. Natural internal dialogue

4. Adequate movement

Our ancestors lived their lives applying these pillars to their lifestyles without even knowing, and lived full, healthy lives. By reading this book you will be able to accomplish the same. You will have the energy and health to live a full and healthy life!

Don't miss out on this opportunity to maximize your health. Start now! Be the person other people look up to as an example. Be that example!

Continue reading to learn more about these four concepts and how to implement them in a holistic manner into your life. You can take control of your own health. Simple, right? Let's do it!

Finding the desire!
The first step in the journey to true health and well-being

Achieving true health and well-being is a way of life. If you want to be well, you must choose this lifestyle. You can't accomplish wellness in a day; it's an ongoing way of life. You must consciously and continually strive for improvement. With time and effort, this lifestyle will become a natural part of your life. However, there is no middle ground. You're either progressing to wellness or regressing to sickness!

This idea may be hard to swallow. Society has become stagnant in so many ways – personal health being one!

Most people run on the hamster wheel of life. They live in brick boxes, drive to work in metal boxes, work in concrete and glass boxes, drive back home in metal boxes, and watch TV boxes. The 8 to 10 hours they spend at their desks each day kill off their inspiration and innovation. When they get home, they only want to sit on their couches and spend their few free hours thinking about nothing (hence, the popularity of junk TV). They buy trendy consumer items to fill this emptiness and go back to work to pay off their credit card balances.

Unfortunately, most people don't seek lifestyle change until they experience a health crisis. Those who neglect their bodies, treat them poorly, and fill them with junk almost always reach a crisis point. They don't make major lifestyle changes because they want to, but because they have to.

Hopefully, you're not in crisis and want to embrace a lifestyle of true health and well-being before things get out of hand. Remember, we're always moving in one direction or the other; toward or away from true health and well-being. Engaging in impulsive actions and "just living life" take you in the wrong direction.

Take a deep breath. Don't worry – no one's perfect.

I recommend the 80/20 rule to all of my patients at the beginning. As you begin to make changes in lifestyle, this strategy makes success feel achievable. The 80/20 rule means reaching your goals 80 percent of the time. If you can eventually get to 95/5, that's even better.

The final goal is to reach 100 percent health and well-being. It is possible and you can achieve it. However, if you make a mistake, don't kick yourself when you slip up; just pick yourself up and keep on going.

The lifestyle I am talking about is difficult to grasp because for generations "sickness care" has been taught, not "health care." People think they're healthy until they feel physical symptoms.

When people feel a symptom like mild pain, they typically take over-the-counter medication. If they feel stronger pains, they go to their doctor looking for a more potent drug.

Have you ever thought about what happens when you take pills?

Yes, pills may make your physical symptoms go away. But, was your problem a lack of medication – or was there another reason for your pain?

People don't ask, "What's the underlying cause of my symptoms?" They want relief without changing their habits or lifestyles. Once their symptoms go away, they return to their normal routines until they feel them again – and the cycle repeats itself.

People aren't at fault for thinking this way; it's how we've been taught for generations. To achieve true health and well-being, you must be willing to make changes in your belief systems and lifestyles. Only after realizing the need for change can you begin your journey forward.

A change in behavior or lifestyle can only come with a change in belief systems. Behaviors, or your lifestyle choices, are the consequence of your belief systems. To find true health and well-being we need to dig deep and change our belief systems, not just a behavior or lifestyle choice.

We can look at our belief systems as our paradigm. Stephen Covey, the author of *7 Habits of Highly Effective People*, has a good explanation of what a paradigm is. He explains that a paradigm is the way one sees the world; it is the lens in which one sees things. It isn't just a shift in beliefs or lifestyle choices, but a shift in paradigms.

It you are willing to change your paradigm of health and apply the four pillars, which I will talk about in more detail, you will establish true health and well-being. But, you must decide to change your health paradigm! You have to commit to changing your way of life – your lifestyle!

You can do it – I'll walk beside you every step of the way. Just keep reading. In the upcoming chapters, I'll expand on this health philosophy.

Who we truly are!

Most people who work within the branches of medicine treat patients in a compartmentalized manner. They treat symptoms or disease or sickness and are not concerned of the true underlying problem. Not because they are not concerned about the health of the patient, but because they are taught to treat symptoms.

Since the infamous Flexner Report of 1910, medicine has always looked to diagnose and treat sickness from the outside using mostly medication or surgery.

Over the last 100 years we have seen an enormous increase in all types of metabolic diseases, examples being diabetes, heart disease, cancers, and autoimmune diseases like rheumatoid arthritis and hypothyroidism to name just a few.

The main reason is because modern medicine looks at human beings as a system of parts instead of a whole system. If we ever want to know what it feels like to be truly well we must understand that we are not just a bunch of separate parts connected together, but an ecosystem of trillions of cells that work harmoniously together to maintain health. Not only are we an ecosystem, but we live on earth, which is an ecosystem that needs to be healthy for us to be healthy. We are an integral part of the ecosystem we call Earth. I did not say we are in control, but part of. What has inevitably happened every time we have tried to take control of nature? A disaster. What happens when we leave nature alone after we have intervened? It returns to its natural and healthy habitat. This is what we must understand first. The less we intervene the better!

An ecosystem is basically a biological community of interacting organisms and their physical environment. True health and wellness comes from the cellular level. Each individual cell in our human body has its role in health, however the way they interact with other cells is much more important.

The question, "How am I going to keep trillions of cells healthy and working harmoniously together so I can feel my best?" might sound daunting and even scary to think about. That is what I love about health. We have the easy part – health is simple! If we provide our bodies with the few basic ingredients I am talking about in this book, our bodies do the rest.

Our bodies not only maintain themselves if we provide the needed ingredients but they will recuperate, they will heal the same way any natural ecosystem does, and they will return to a healthy natural state. I once read a great quote from physician, educator, and researcher Lewis Thomas who said,

> "The great secret of medicine, known to doctors but still hidden from the public, is that most things get better by themselves."

This quote contains many truths to it. However it is missing the importance of finding true health and wellness, by providing our bodies with the few ingredients it requires to reach true health, which is an ecosystem of cells working harmoniously together.

What you must understand is that you are incredibly powerful. You, reading this right now, are incredibly powerful, and you have the capacity to heal yourself. To hear that we have control of our health could be one of the most liberating and also one of the most terrifying thoughts we might have. It implies that we must take responsibility for our health, and must never leave our health in the hands of others.

So who are we truly? We are an ecosystem of trillions of cells that work harmoniously together. We have the potential to self heal and self regulate. Our bodies are much more intelligent than we were taught, and even understand. If we give our bodies a few vital ingredients, our bodies will do the rest. We do not even need to worry about symptoms; our bodies know best, and we must trust them.

Nutrient dense food
Gut health and its importance

Over the years the importance of gut health has become very clear in its role in our overall health and well-being. The gut, our digestive system, plays a huge role in our physical and mental well-being. The importance of eating nutrient dense food that comes from fertile soil without chemicals is one of the vital pillars to true health and well-being. It is much more important today than ever!

The main reason why I started Pastos Verdes Farm with my family was to provide our family food that is nutrient dense. We started the farm raising chicken for meat. We did this because meat is a food that has become very contaminated and toxic over the years with the introduction of Concentrated Animal Feeding Operation (CAFO) farms.

Before I talk about the problem with our food system, I need to explain that it is not due to the farmers. The farmers have been put between a rock and a hard place. They also need to make a living, and with all the government subsidies and low profit margin, they are forced to continually expand their farms. With each expansion, they must invest in more land, more equipment, and they accrue more debt. Between the hybrid GMO (genetically modified organism) seed from Monsanto and the government subsidies that completely destroy the ability of the free market to function, the farmers have a very hard time making enough to provide for their own families. Farmers are doing the best they can with the situation that has been given to them. However, there are some great farmers out there like Will Harris III of White Oak Pastures in Bluffton, Georgia that are making positive changes, and he's not alone. More and more family farms are starting up and providing local nutrient dense food, grown or raised on fertile soil without chemicals, like Primal Pastures in Southern California and Polyface Farms in West Virginia. Farms like these, and many more like them, are meeting the demand for nutrient dense food!

Meat – one of the important components of our diet.

In CAFO farms, the animals are raised in an area where they don't have much room to even move! They live the majority of their lives in their own excrement! This isn't just done with chickens but also with pigs, cows, and any other type of meat that is found in the supermarket.

In chicken CAFO farms – which we could really call a factory, where the numbers range between 10,000 and 50,000 – chickens live packed into a hoop house that is completely closed off. Yes, you read that right – up to 50,000 chickens in one single hoop house! They practically never see the light of day, they move very little, and are fed grains full of chemicals twenty-four hours a day. They never see a blade of grass! During their short lives of five to six weeks they are also given antibiotics to fight off the many infections they pick up from breathing all the excrement particles in the hazy air inside the hoop house. Now, chicken producers are not allowed to give these chickens hormones to help in growth. The way they get around this is by injecting the hormone into the egg a couple days before the chicken hatches. Without the hormones, their bones would break under their own weight due to the incredibly rapid rate of growth. What you have before they are shipped off for processing is a sick bird full of antibiotics, hormones, and toxins like arsenic, which is a known neurotoxin.

The butchering process is just as awful. These chickens grow so fast that at five to six weeks they are transported in huge tractor trailers to where they are butchered. The transportation causes a huge amount of stress on the chickens that are already stressed to an unbelievable point. At the processing plant, about 170 birds are processed a minute. Yes, you read that right, too – 170 a minute! They are first shocked, then killed. Then all the offal, or organs, is sucked out. The organs of a healthy bird can be very nutritious, but for these birds, they have to be thrown out due to the high amount of toxins found in them. With the suctioning of the offal, many times the intestines rupture causing excrement to spray all over the toxin rich bird. To prevent contamination, most birds are washed in chlorine baths up to thirty times. The chicken is then packaged and packed into huge refrigerated trailers and shipped usually thousands of miles to a supermarket near you, where you go and buy that bird and cook it and feed it to your family. I use chickens as an example because that is exactly what we raise on Pastos Verdes Farm. Just like chickens, all other animals at CAFO farms are treated the same. Ruminant animals like the cow, which are animals with four stomachs, require a diet of grass, but they are given the same diet as a chicken, grains!

We have become so accustomed to this form of meat that when we see marbled meat from a cow we think we are eating the best type of meat, which is the complete opposite of what is true. We are eating flesh filled with saturated fat spread throughout the whole muscle. When we eat meat, the fat should be on the outside of the muscle!

It is so important that we educate ourselves about the current food system because what you are reading will never be found in mainstream media. It is so important to understand what is going on with the current food system!

With this type of system, we see more and more people not eating meat. They see how these animals are treated and can't support a system so cruel. I completely understand their point of view as a humanitarian, however, with respect to proper nutrition, I cannot see a diet without meat as being complete.

What needs to be done is help people understand that there are places where animals are raised in a proper manner, and in safe locations where they can enjoy a full and satisfying life. I love how fellow farmer and author, Joel Salatin explains it when he says a chicken needs to live a life of a chicken, a pig needs to live a life of a pig, and a cow needs to live a life of a cow. If we find farmers that do just that we can be sure that our meat will be full of the nutrients our bodies need to function in a healthy manner.

On our farm, we do it right, and we will do it right again when we start up our farm in Argentina. We give our chickens a life of a chicken – they live outside with the sun and sky above them, so they have all the vitamin D and fresh air necessary. They have grass and bugs below them, so they get all the other vitamins, minerals and protein necessary. They have room to run around, scratch, play, dig, bathe, and live a lovely life of a chicken. We supplement their grass and bugs with organic non-GMO feed and also supply clean well water for their drinking.

My favorite part of the day while farming is the mornings, when I go move the portable dome coop and give the chickens a new fresh salad to munch on. Seeing them race around, first looking for bugs and then calming down and just eating grass, is a sight everybody should experience.

I love the new trend small local farms are starting of giving farm tours. There isn't a better way to find good, locally grown food. You not only get to know your farmer but have the opportunity to get out in nature and enjoy the natural beauty of this earth and the clean fresh air. Something we all need a lot more of.

The processing of our chickens is just as humane as their life. We process at eight weeks. We also process on farm. I transport our chickens, five at a time, about 150 feet. There is absolutely no transportation stress and their life is also practically stress-free. This means there will be no stress hormone in the meat. I personally, and with the help of others, slit the throat the proper way at a 45-degree angle below the beak right at the jugular vein, sharpening the knife each time to make sure there is a clean cut.

Unfortunately, I have personal experience with what a clean cut feels like. While I worked as a carpenter to get through school I accidentally cut myself with a freshly sharpened hatchet. The cut was so deep that it went all the way through to the fascia. If I hadn't looked down and seen the thick and deep cut, I would have never known I had cut myself. I felt absolutely nothing! I now have a beautiful scar on my right forearm as a result of that day!

We then pluck and clean the birds ourselves with no suctioning. We remove the offal, taking the stomach, liver, and heart, and save them for consumption. These organs are rich with nutrients! We also save the feet for use in chicken broth. We use very little water, and all other parts of the birds are composted to further enrich the soil where the grass is growing so the birds get the most nutritious grass possible.

It can be a beautiful process where everybody wins – the animal lives a wonderful life, we as humans get the nutrition that our bodies ask for, and everything else goes back into the soil to further enrich the animals' food. It is a win-win-win situation!

Vegetables and fruits – important components of our diet.

Vegetables are probably the most important component of our diets and should be the majority of our diet. Just like with meat, modern industrial farming practices, with respect to vegetables and fruits, are causing havoc on our health. Today we don't see a lot of small local farms growing food for their community. In the United States, 2 percent of the population grow the food for the other 98 percent. Those are insane numbers! Those numbers make it impossible to grow food in a manner that does not destroy the soil in which the food is grown.

That is the first problem with the vegetables! The majority of people are consuming vegetables that come from soils that are literally dead. It is dirt, nothing more! These vegetables come from what are called monocrop farms. These are farms where one crop is grown on hundreds to thousands of acres.

When the United States was expanding, the farmers would work the land until it wouldn't produce anymore. They would then leave the land and find another piece of land that was fertile, usually cutting down many trees in the process, and would farm that piece of land. This happened over and over again as the farmers moved more and more west. Farms today work a little differently. Instead of moving on to a new piece of land, they use chemical fertilizers to keep their plants alive. Chemists found that plants only need three elements to survive. "Survive" is the proper word because they are definitely not thriving. Those three elements are nitrogen, phosphorus, and potassium. They formulated a chemical substance with these three elements and now farmers, with a chemical spray, can keep their plants alive until they harvest a very nutrient-poor crop.

Not only are chemical fertilizers used but chemical pesticides and herbicides as well, because the plants themselves are too weak to fight off pests and become overpowered by bugs and weeds. Really, we need to call them as they really are, they are poisons!

We are also seeing more and more GMO seeds. It is difficult to believe that scientists are taking genes from other organisms and inserting them into the seeds of plants that we are consuming. How far from nature have we come? It is scary at times! The reason they have to fabricate these seeds is to make them resilient enough to handle the increasingly strong pesticides and herbicides being used. With the use of pesticides, we are making pesticide-resistant pests, and with herbicides, we are making herbicide-resistant weeds. It makes sense – with herbicide you are killing off all the weaker weeds, leaving the stronger weeds to reproduce, and each generation is more and more resistant to the herbicide. The same happens with pesticides. The weak bugs are killed off, leaving the stronger bugs to not only reproduce, but become more and more resistant to all pesticides. Now, farmers are having more and more difficulty keeping a crop pest and weed free. It is a cycle that we cannot win, because nature always wins. To be able to feed the world with nutrient dense food we must work with nature, not against it!

Fats and oils – not to be scared of. Our bodies need them!

First things first – the difference in fats!

Saturated fats are fats that cannot hold any more hydrogen. They are completely full of hydrogen and are found mostly in animal meats.

Animals raised in CAFO farms are high in saturated fats, while animals raised properly have a lot less saturated fat. With grain-only fed beef, a paltry 1 percent of the fat is omega-3, a fat that we must provide our bodies. However, omega-3's in beef raised on grass account for 7 percent of the total fat content.

 Ruminant animals, like cows, goats, and sheep, need to eat grass, not grains. When they are raised this way, the fat is located outside the muscle, and overall there is a lot less saturated fat.

The recommended ratio of omega-6 to omega-3 fatty acids in humans is 3:1 to 1:1. The ratio in beef raised on grass is 3:1, or in other words, when we eat beef raised properly we get the recommended ratio of omega-6 and omega-3.

Unsaturated fat is a fat or fatty acid in which there is at least one double bond within the fatty acid chain. A fatty acid chain is monounsaturated if it contains one double bond, and polyunsaturated if it contains more than one double bond.

Some food sources of monounsaturated fats include:

- olive oil
- canola oil
- peanut oil
- nuts
- avocados

Polyunsaturated fats can be divided into two main groups known as omega-3 fats and omega-6 fats. There are other omega fatty acids like omega-9, however they are not talked about as much because they are not essential. In other words, we can create these fatty acids, so we don't need to get them from our food.

Omega-3 fats include:

- oily fish such as salmon and sardines
- eggs and meats that are raised properly
- plant sources including flaxseed, walnuts, green leafy vegetables (lettuce, broccoli, kale, spinach, etc.)
- legumes (kidney, navy, pinto or lima beans, peas or split peas, etc.)

- citrus fruits, melons, cherries.

Animal sources of omega-3 have been shown to have more benefits for cardiovascular health than plant sources of omega-3.

Omega-6 fats include:

- sunflower, soybean, sesame oils
- nuts (such as walnuts, pecans, brazil and pine nuts)
- sunflower seeds

Then there are the trans fats. The artificial or chemically prepared trans fat is what causes the majority of problems.

What are trans fats?

In chemical terms, *trans fat* is a fat molecule that contains one or more double bonds in trans geometric configuration. A double bond may exhibit one of two possible configurations: *trans* or *cis*. The *trans* molecule is a straight molecule. The *cis* molecule is bent.

There are two types of trans fats found in foods: naturally occurring and artificial trans fats. Naturally occurring trans fats are produced in the gut of some animals, and foods made from these animals – for example milk and meat products – may contain small quantities of these fats. Artificial trans fats or trans fatty acids are created in an industrial process that adds hydrogen to liquid vegetable oils in order to make them more solid.

Trans vaccenic acid, a natural animal trans fat found in dairy and beef products, can actually reduce risk factors associated with heart disease, diabetes, and obesity, according to a researcher from the University of Alberta[1].

The benefit was due in part to the ability of vaccenic acid to reduce the production of chylomicrons, which are particles of fat and cholesterol that form in your small intestine following a meal. They are then rapidly processed throughout the body, and may be related to a variety of conditions arising from metabolic disorders.

Experiments on rats showed that vaccenic acid in the diet could lower total cholesterol by approximately 30 percent, LDL cholesterol by 25 percent, and triglyceride levels by more than 50 percent.

Here we see nature at its best. By consuming a fat that comes from a properly raised animal we see the exact opposite of what most people think of fat. It decreases cholesterol!

Artificial trans fat is what we want to avoid. However, these fats are found everywhere because they are easy to use, inexpensive to produce, and don't go bad. Many restaurants and fast food outlets also use artificial trans fats to deep-fry foods because oils with artificial trans fats can be used many times in commercial fryers.

Trans fats are found in fried foods like doughnuts and baked goods, including cakes, pie crusts, biscuits, frozen pizza, cookies, crackers, stick margarines and other spreads. You can determine the amount of artificial trans fats in a particular packaged food by looking at the Nutrition Facts panel. However, products can be listed as "0 grams of trans fats" if they contain 0 grams to less than 0.5 grams of artificial trans fat per serving. You can also spot artificial trans fats by reading ingredient lists and looking for the ingredients referred to as "partially hydrogenated oils."

Not only is the modern diet toxic with artificial trans fats but the modern diet is dangerously deficient in omega-3 fatty acids.

The imbalance in today's modern day diet of the omega-6 to omega-3 ratio is between 15:1 and 17:1. Remember, the ideal fatty acid ratio should range from 3:1 to 1:1. This imbalance has severe health implications.

These fatty acids, the omega-3's and omega-6's, are a major part of the cell membrane. The cell membrane is like a cell's gatekeeper. It's the outer layer that surrounds a cell, letting substances in or keeping them out.

You can think of a cell membrane as a rubber membrane that keeps rain from seeping through your roof; it surrounds and protects the contents of a cell. It controls which substances can enter and exit the cell. The membrane also gives a cell its shape and enables the cell to attach to other cells, forming tissues. In other words, the cell membrane is very important!

Fatty acids help keep the membrane of the cell fluid and permeable so the right nutrients are able to enter the cell. To keep our cells healthy we need these fatty acids.

There are three omega-3 fatty acids that are especially important in the development of our nervous system. Our nervous system being what controls everything we do consciously and subconsciously. These three omega-3 fatty acids are EPA (Eicosapentaenoic acid), AA (Arachidonic acid) and especially DHA (Docosahexaenoic acid). These omega-3's are only found in wild game or properly raised meats and fish. Our body is designed to consume these fatty acids, not convert all of them from another fatty acid that comes from plants.

The book *The Innate Diet & Natural Hygiene* by James Chestnut, D.C. gives an excellent illustration that I would like to share about the importance of getting these omega fatty acids.

> "Imagine your brain conducting some routine maintenance on your dopamine and serotonin receptors (implicated in both ADD and mood disorders.) These receptors are composed of an omega 3 fatty acid called DHA. If you don't have much DHA in your blood, man-made trans fat molecules may be used as a construction material instead. But trans fats are shaped differently than DHA; they are straight while DHA is curved. The dopamine receptor becomes deformed and doesn't work very well. Repeat this scenario day

after day, year after year and you could wind up with problems like depression and problems concentrating. This problem is most severe for a child whose brain is still developing. A lack of highly unsaturated fats is particularly noticeable in connections with brain and nerve function. An adjustment in diet to one with oil and protein contents high in unsaturated fats brings the best results in children."

"Now imagine a child in school learning math. The act of learning requires the brain to form new neural pathways. DHA is needed, especially for the delicate neural synapses, which are composed entirely of DHA. This child, like the vast majority of US children, eats almost no omega 3 fatty acids. What does the brain do? Again, it struggles and finally uses other types of fats, which are the wrong shape. The neural network develops slowly and is defective. The child has learning and memory problems as well as behavior problems."

Omega-3's and omega-6's are found in both plants and in animals. However, different omega-3's are found in plant-based foods and others are found in animal-based foods.

Remember those three polyunsaturated fats that I talked about that are so important in the development of your nervous system. Those three omega-3 fatty acids make up about 94 percent of all the polyunsaturated fats that are found in the gray matter of the brain. These three polyunsaturated fats are found in meats. Yes, it has been shown that other polyunsaturated fats can be converted into these other important fats, however it has been shown that they are too slow to provide a sufficient supply during early human brain development. It is very important that we supply them.

The human brain is more than 60 percent structural fat, just as our muscles are made of protein and our bones are made of calcium. It is not just any fat that our brains are made of. It has to be certain types of fats. We no longer eat these types of fats like we used to. Worse, we eat artificial trans fats and excessive amounts of saturated fats and vegetable oils.

That is why fats and oils, which is just a liquid fat, get such a bad name. So many people stop eating fats because they think all fat is unhealthy. The truth is that the only fat we must avoid at all cost is artificial trans fats. Most people need to increase the amount of fats they are consuming, not decrease them.

Grains – the one food source we should be eating less of!

The majority of our ancestors lived on a diet that provided all the nutrition their bodies required. Their diets had an average ratio of 65 percent plant to 35 percent animal. Most of the plants consumed were vegetables with very little grains because of the amount of work it took to get one grain. These days, with all the machinery we have, it is easy to get wheat. But sadly, it's not easy to get properly raised grains. The reality for the health-conscious consumer is that almost all supermarket flour is made from industrial modern wheat, and almost all of it is made with industrial processing.

Have you ever wondered how a wheat berry becomes modern-day processed flour? Or how white flour is made?

Most commercial wheat production, unfortunately, begins with the seeds being treated with fungicides. Once they become wheat, they are sprayed with hormones and pesticides and herbicides. Even the bins in which the harvested wheat is stored have been coated with insecticides. If bugs appear on the wheat in storage, they again fumigate the grain. We are eating a seed that has been sprayed and sprayed and sprayed with chemicals. Does that worry you just a little bit?

A whole grain of wheat, sometimes called a wheat berry, is composed of three layers:

- the bran
- the germ
- the endosperm

The bran is the hard outer shell of the kernel, and it's the layer where you'll find most of the fiber. The germ is the nutrient-rich embryo that will sprout into a new wheat plant. The endosperm is the largest part of the grain, making up 83 percent of the kernel, and it's mostly starch.

White flour is made from the endosperm only, whereas whole wheat flour combines all three parts of the wheat berry.

Old time mills ground flour slowly, but today's mills are designed for mass-production, using high-temperature, high-speed steel rollers. The resulting white flour is nearly all starch, and even much of today's commercially processed whole wheat flour has lost a fair amount of nutritional value due to these aggressive processing methods.

The processing of wheat started in the 1870's, when the invention of the modern steel roller mill revolutionized grain milling. Compared to old stone methods, it was fast and efficient and gave fine control over the various parts of the kernel. Instead of just mashing it all together, one could separate the component parts, allowing the purest and finest of white flour to be easily produced at low cost. This new type of flour shipped and stored better, allowing for a long distribution chain. In fact, it kept almost indefinitely. Pest problems were practically eliminated because pests didn't want it. Of course, we now know that the reason it keeps so well is that it has been stripped of vital nutrients. The bugs and rodents knew this way before we did.

The steel roller mill became so popular, so fast, that within ten years nearly all stone mills in the western world had been replaced. As a result, the first processed food and the beginning of our industrial food system was born, where vast quantities of shelf-stable "food" is produced in large factories, many months and many miles from the point of consumption.

While these "advances" in milling were hailed as an innovation of modern living, nobody thought much about what was happening to the actual food value of wheat. Even worse is that for decades now the health problems due to industrial white flour have been known and industrial white flour is still, by far, the most popular way to eat wheat.

But there is another, newer, problem caused by a second technology revolution in the 20th century. It is not nearly as widely understood, but this "advancement" in farming and food production may have wrecked wheat itself.

The world's wheat crop was transformed in the 1950's and 1960's in a movement called the "Green Revolution." The father of the movement, Norman Borlaug, was awarded the Nobel Peace Prize, and credited with saving one billion lives. Borlaug led teams that looked to develop high-yielding varieties of cereal grains. They also worked on the expansion of irrigation infrastructure, modernization of management techniques, distribution of hybridized seeds, and synthetic fertilizers and pesticides to farmers.

He pioneered new species of semi-dwarf wheat that, together with fertilizers and pesticides, increased yield enormously. This new farming technology was propagated around the world by companies like Dupont and Monsanto. Like the industrial milling revolution before it, the green revolution applied new technologies to improve efficiency and output, with little or no regard to the effect on human nutrition. We are now discovering many of the unintended consequences of this Green Revolution.

According to Wheat Belly author Dr. William Davis,

> "this thing being sold to us called wheat – it ain't wheat. It's this stocky, little, high-yield plant, a distant relative of the wheat our mothers used to bake muffins, genetically and biochemically light-years removed from the wheat of just 40 years ago."

And now there are connections between the chemical laced modern wheat and all manner of chronic digestive and inflammatory illnesses.

For thousands of years, wheat has been cultivated, stored, milled and consumed. The system worked, and it helped in the nourishment of some populations. In the last 150 years we decided to change things.

First, the mechanical technologies that turned wheat into barren white flour; then, the chemical and genetic technologies to make it easier to harvest and resistant to pests, drought, and blight.

What we really have are mutant seeds, grown in synthetic soil, bathed in chemicals. They're deconstructed, pulverized to fine dust, bleached and chemically treated to create a barren industrial filler that no other creature on the planet will eat. And we wonder why it might be making us sick?

The simple and obvious solution is don't eat wheat. That's why we have the gluten-free craze. But for most of us there is an alternative solution: don't eat industrial flour made with modern wheat.

If we are going to eat wheat we need to return to honest to goodness, old fashioned flour: heirloom wheats, like Einkorn berries, Red Fife berries or Spelt and Kamut berries, freshly stone ground. The best way to get fresh wholesome flour is to buy yourself a countertop grain mill, find an heirloom wheat, and mill it yourself, as you need it. The quality is amazing and you will be thrilled with the results.

The answer to the modern food system!

I know you are thinking, "Well what in the world am I supposed to do now? The modern food system has turned food into a product that has no nutritional value!"

However, there is a great example out there that gives us the answers to all our nutritional needs. There are people, just like you, that lived a full life and got all the proper nutrition their bodies required. Our ancestors! Many of us don't even need to go back many generations to find the lifestyle where all nutrition was provided in the proper amount.

If we look to them using today's technology there is absolutely no reason why we cannot provide our bodies with the required nutrition to function at its best, and truly be well.

I love the quote made by one of my favorite regenerative farmers, Joel Salatin:

> "The first supermarket supposedly appeared on the American landscape in 1946. That is not very long ago. Until then, where was all the food? Dear folks, the food was in homes, gardens, local fields, and forests. It was near kitchens, near tables, near bedsides. It was in the pantry, the cellar, the backyard."

1946? That was just seventy years ago. Most of us have grandparents that were alive seventy years ago! Most of us still have access to the knowledge needed to provide our bodies with the necessary nutrition. What an opportunity! If you are lucky enough to still have your grandparents, or even some of you your great grandparents, the first thing you should be doing is asking them how they lived when they were young. Not only asking them, but using today's technology and recording the conversations.

This is exactly how it was done in the past. The elderly, with all their knowledge, focused on bringing up the following generations. There was no need for medical schools or degrees in nutrition. The medical schools and nutrition majors were in the minds of the elderly who would pass that information on to the next generation. All the medicinal herbs that were used to prevent and cure were known not by reading the latest text book and then taking a multiple choice test like how I did it, but by the elderly in the community. The techniques to grow and find nutrient dense food was taught by those with experience. The elderly had their role in the community, not like in today's society where the majority of the elderly are in nursing homes. They were the most respected and sought after knowledge that there was.

Let's start our journey to finding nutrient dense food by bringing that one very important aspect of life back. Let's let our ancestors teach us, which is their primary role! They might not know how to use the current iPhone, but most do know what is really important. Like how to plant a garden, what herbs are used for different ailments, the concepts of frugality, and how to live a simple but satisfying life. Most understand how to live healthier lives because they lived it not too many years ago.

That is step one, and many times one of the most satisfying steps. Getting to know your grandparents, or if you are lucky enough your great grandparents, is not only knowledgeable, but learning about your family history is one of the most interesting things you will learn in your personal life!

Running outside with the shovel and planting a garden is the second step. But first, get to know your own roots, and nourish them. Then, plant the seeds that will eventually leave new roots, and will in turn bring you the proper nutrition in balance your body needs.

Planting a garden is the absolute best method of giving yourself and your family the proper nutrition in balance. There are many ways to garden, however if you have never gardened before in your life, I recommend Mel Bartholomew's square foot garden method. Once you start to see the results and taste the incredible things you grew yourself, there is no going back!

From all my studies on how to farm better, I came across a design system that has completely revolutionized the way we farm. This method is nothing new, but what it has done is bring many methods into one, making a system that is complete. A system that not only gives you nutrient dense food but also builds soil in the process. This system is called permaculture.

Permaculture – grow food and build soil at the same time!

Permaculture was termed by its founders, Bill Mollison and David Holmgren. It is the combination of the words "permanent" and "agriculture," however permaculture has evolved to a system where it builds regenerative cultures. The word "culture" comes from the Latin *cultura*, and from the French *culture*, both of which mean "care for, till, place tilled and honor."

We all have our culture. I happen to have two. My dad was born in the United States and was raised in the North American culture, while my mother, born in Argentina, was raised with the Argentine culture. Luckily I got the two combined! It doesn't matter where we are born or what culture we live in, each and every one of our cultures begins with the caring of earth. That is the first ethic of permaculture. Care of earth is what brings about all life. There is a cycle of life where everything begins and ends in the soil of the planet. If we want to be healthy we must have healthy soil. Permaculture teaches many methods of how to build soil and grow nutrient dense food at the same time.

As we care for the earth and build soil, the other two ethics of permaculture come naturally. These are the care of people and a return of surplus, which is the return of extra energy back into the systems that care for the land and the people.

To sum it up, permaculture has three ethics:

- care of earth
- care of people
- return of surplus

These three ethics build on each other. Everything that is done in permaculture cares for earth and people, and builds systems that are sustainable and regenerative.

This is done by using systems of design involving the six growing zones, which build efficient energy use and the seven layers of growth found in nature – something I will expand upon in a moment. By using these zones and layers we build systems where one component of the garden will have many jobs, otherwise known as "stacking functions," which is a common term used in permaculture. Take the chicken for example. A chicken not only gives us a highly nutritious food, but it also scratches the ground, eats the grass, and leaves droppings, preparing the ground for the next round of plants.

In permaculture, when you plan on how you will design your food system you use zones to be as efficient with energy usage as possible. This ranges from the amount of energy you exert to how much energy your house will consume. The six zones include:

Zone 0 – This is your home. Here permaculture principles are used to reduce energy and water needs. This is done by using all the natural resources available to us such as sunlight, and rain. We do this to create a harmonious, sustainable environment in which to live, work, and relax.

Zone 1 – This is the zone nearest to your home, This is where you plant what needs the most attention like all your salad greens and other annual vegetables (vegetables that die at first frost), herbs, soft fruit like strawberries or raspberries. Here you can also place a small greenhouse used as an area to start seeds and worm compost bin for kitchen waste.

Zone 2 – This area is used for perennial plants (plants that survive a frost) that require less frequent maintenance. For example, occasional weeding using natural methods like mulching, and pruning. This area can include fruiting bushes and orchards. Here you also see beehives and larger scale compost bins.

Zone 3 – This is the area where you grow your main crops. This being your main calorie crops like nuts and meats, this also includes seed crops like rice. Here is where you also start to grow for trade purposes. After establishment, care and maintenance required is low.

Zone 4 – Is semi-wild. This zone is mainly used for forage and collecting wild food. This area is where you also can grow trees for building material.

Zone 5 – This is untouched land. There is no human intervention in this area apart from observation of the natural ecosystems and their cycles. Zone 5 is where we continually learn the important lesson in permaculture of working with nature, not against it.

With the six zones in place, the plan comes together using the seven canopy layers.

The first layer is the Canopy or Tall Tree Layer, which is really only used in larger designs. Here we see tall trees, large nut trees, timber trees, and larger fruiting trees.

The second layer is called the Sub-Canopy Layer or the Large Shrub Layer. This is the starting layer when you have limited space. These plants often make up the acting canopy layer. The majority of the fruit trees are found in this layer.

The third layer is the Shrub Layer. This is where we find the majority of fruiting bushes. This layer also includes many nut plants, flowering plants, medicinal plants, and other beneficial plants.

The fourth layer is called the Herbaceous Layer. This is the layer where the plants die back to the ground every winter, if winters are cold enough. The plants do not produce woody stems as the Shrub Layer does. In this layer we find many of the culinary and medicinal herbs.

The fifth layer is the Groundcover Layer. Here we see some overlap with the Herbaceous Layer. The difference is in this layer the plants are more shade tolerant, grow much closer to the ground, grow densely to fill bare patches of soil, and can often tolerate some foot traffic.

The sixth layer is the Underground Layer. Here we find all the root crops. There is a huge variety of edible roots that most people have never heard of.

The last layer is called the Vertical Layer. In this layer you find all the vining and climbing plants which climb into the first six layers. This is where we can add more productivity to a small space.

Using the six zones and the seven layers found in nature, the beginning of a beautiful space where an abundance of nutrient dense food can be grown is started. Permaculture is not only found in areas with lots of land. By understanding the zones and layers, and using other permaculture principles, you can even grow a lot of your own food on your balcony. Don't let space be your crutch. There are many ways to grow food even in small areas.

Where do I find food that is nutrient dense?

In a lifestyle of wellness the first place you will find some of the nutrient dense food your body requires is in your own backyard. It is important to grow some of our food. It can be 1 percent of what we consume, but the process of planting a seed and eating the food that comes from that plant is very important. There are various reasons why. First, we become part of the great cycle of life. We get to see the birth of a seed, we get to nurture it through its life and enjoy the food that comes from it, and then compost that plant to help the next plant be as healthy as possible. Second, the food we are consuming is the freshest possible. The fresher the food we consume the more nutritious it will be. There is nothing more fresh than walking outside, harvesting, and walking back inside to eat. Third, we know exactly what went into the food we are consuming. We know that if the seed is a good seed, and that no chemicals were used, we can be certain we are eating a highly nutritious food. Fourth, working the land and growing plants psychologically heals us. And fifth, working in fertile soil physiologically heals us. It has been found that fertile soil contains a bacterium called *mycobacterium vacaue*, which triggers the secretion of serotonin, a hormone that elevates mood and helps decrease the now famous stress hormones cortisol and the Catecholamines.

The second place you will find nutrient dense food is your local farms. We need to get to know our farmers. Most of us are not going to grow and raise 100 percent of our food. Many of us just don't have the space to do it. However, that is not an excuse. I have interviewed people on my podcast(2) living in cities who have grown the majority of their food. The food we do not grow or raise ourselves must come from a source we know. The more personal the relationship the better. It isn't just buying organic anymore! We need to know where our food is coming from. This means that you actually visit the farm, which is one important step. If the farmer allows you to see his operation, you'll be sure that he is doing a lot of things right. Buying as local and in season as possible is another important step. Most food that is not grown in your own backyard can now be found elsewhere locally. It is becoming easier and easier to find locally grown food that is properly grown or raised. Many times a simple internet search will turn up farms in your area that provide naturally-raised food. There are also great websites that are helping the consumer find the farmer like http://www.eatwild.com.

The third place to find nutrient dense food, and only when we cannot grow it ourselves or source it locally, is the local supermarket. If we are going to buy in a supermarket the word 'organic' does still play an important role. Don't buy the cheapest product. It is scary how most people will research the best televisions on the market and be willing to pay more for a name brand, but when it comes to the food we consume – one of the most important decisions we make various times a day – we settle for the cheapest product out there. Just like we study out the best television, we must do the same with the food we purchase at the supermarket. Don't buy the cheapest product; study the different brands and make sure you are buying a product that won't do you harm!

When we buy from a supermarket we want to avoid the center aisles, which are filled with all the processed foods. The foods we do buy from a supermarket usually come from farms that are thousands of miles away, if not from a different country entirely. The freshness is lost and much of the nutrition our bodies require is not present.

Many say that nutrient dense food is expensive. If all we are doing is buying from a supermarket, yes, it will be more expensive. That is yet another reason why it is so important to grow as much of our own food as possible – it is just cheaper that way. But if it is not possible, the hard truth is we truly cannot afford *not* to consume these foods because our health depends on it.

The reason why we must eat food that is grown or raised properly, the reason why we must grow as much of our food as possible or source it from local farmers that we personally know, is because *our health depends on it.*

Our health depends on a diet of whole foods. It simply comes down to one thing: mother nature knows best. We are an animal species that is genetically adapted to a certain diet. Yet, just in the last 150 years, we have gotten away from traditional foods. It is becoming more and more clear that chronic health and obesity problems around the world are a result of this modern, dysfunctional new diet. It also seems pretty clear now that the closer we stay to a fresh, natural diet, the better. It's simply what our bodies expect, and need, to be healthy, vital, and strong. Yet, we are lacking in essential fatty acids, like omega-3's, and wholesome, unaltered grains, such as modern wheat, which, converted into industrial white flour, is about as far from wholesome as can be imagined. No wonder our bodies are protesting.

We need to eliminate the profound changes in modern wheat, in support of traditional stone-ground flour, milled fresh, with all the nourishment of the living seed intact – a species our bodies will recognize. We need to eliminate the chemical fertilizers, herbicides, fungicides and pesticides of modern industrial farming in support of beyond organic farming and clean seed.

Our modern food system has made being healthy a lot more difficult than it needs to be. Our ancestors didn't know how much of each nutrient our bodies needed. They didn't even know what a supplement was. They didn't know when to eat certain foods. Our ancestors grew and raised some of their food, and some of them *all* of their food. The food they didn't grow themselves they got locally from other farmers. They ate in season and preserved food in ways that preserved the nutrition or even enhanced the nutritional content, like fermentation. Where did all this knowledge of how to grow their own food, prepare nutritious meals using food in season, and preserve food come from? The valued elderly of these communities!

Let's take the first step in regaining our natural health by taking advantage of all the great knowledge of our parents, grandparents, and if you are so lucky your great grandparents. If you do this, you will be one step closer to living the lifestyle of true health. You will be one step closer to living the lifestyle of wellness!

(1) https://academic.oup.com/jn/article/139/11/2049/4751044

(2) http://pastosverdesfarm.libsyn.com/health-permaculture-and-sustainability-all-with-mike-haydon-103

Chiropractic Care
The forgotten pillar

I have a lot of history in the state of Utah. In the 1850's, my ancestors left northern Utah and established a ranch in the southern Utah area now known as Pinto. For many years, the ranch was known as the Old Page Ranch. The Old Page Ranch has a house that still exists and is now a historic monument.

The house took two years to build. On Christmas day, 1900, my great, great-grandfather, Daniel Richie Page, moved his family into the house. My great-grandfather, John Geary Page, spent his youth at the Old Page Ranch House. In the early 1900's, the ranch house was on one of the main roads leading further west and served as a hotel. When it was built, Daniel Richie Page sent one of his sons to Chicago by train with cattle to sell. With the money from the sale of the cattle, he bought furniture, carpets, and wallpaper for the house. This house is a beautiful home!

When I was young, our family had a reunion at the old ranch. I got to know the house and its surroundings but couldn't go inside. I remember the lake in the yard and the beautiful, two-story, red brick house. It's one of the most beautiful sights I remember from my youth. Recently, now married and with two kids, I was able to return to the Old Page Ranch House with my wife and my daughter, Verena. I never imagined what would happen next.

When we got to the house, there were about fifteen people out back with their trucks. That saddened me because we had gone there to get away from everything and enjoy our favorite drink, yerba mate. However, I wasn't going to waste the opportunity to show my wife and daughter the old house. I got out of our truck and showed my daughter a mural that gave a little history of the house. I pointed out my ancestors' names while my wife took pictures.

While I was reading to my daughter, a woman came around the side of the house to get something out of her car. I introduced myself and said I was a descendent of Daniel Richie Page. She put on a big smile and said, "Me, too!" She explained her group was cleaning and winterizing the house. She said we were lucky to visit that day because they were boarding up the windows and doors; soon, no one would be able to see inside. She took us around back and introduced us to everybody. And then the best thing happened – she gave us a tour of the Old Page Ranch House. It was amazing to see the beauty of the house's interior for the first time. I reflected on my ancestors; I was inspired to talk with my grandfather about his father, John Geary Page.

I woke up the next morning and visited my grandfather's home. We talked about what a hard worker my great-grandfather was, and how he could build homes with the best of them.

He described how John raised cattle and grew watermelons at the ranch. However, what really interested me was my great-grandfather's journey to become a chiropractor.

My great-grandfather attended Palmer College of Chiropractic in the 1920's, when the profession was new. I was very interested in this part of his history because I attended the same college. I asked many questions, and my grandfather answered the best he could. I wanted to know why my great-grandfather became a chiropractor. My grandfather told me his father had always wanted to help others. He thought medicine was the best way to help people, but he didn't like the direction modern medicine was going at that time. Incredible! This was in the 1920's!

My great-grandfather decided the best path for him was to go to chiropractic college and become a chiropractor. In 2007, four generations later, his great-grandson (me!) attended the same school for the same reasons. My thought process mirrored my great-grandfather's. I have always wanted to help people; I once thought the medical field was the best way to do this. However, like my great-grandfather, I didn't approve of the direction modern medicine was going. I became a doctor of chiropractic because I knew I could help people find wellness and health by treating them in the chiropractic paradigm. Unfortunately, over the years, many chiropractors (wanting to be accepted by medical doctors) have forgotten the true healing potential of chiropractic.

Most of my conversations about chiropractic resemble one I had not too long ago:

I sat with a group of people in a class while the person in charge introduced the new people to the other members of the group. When it was my turn, the leader told the group I was a chiropractor and said that if anybody had back pain, they knew whom to call. The people in the group started joking around, saying it would be nice to end the class twenty minutes early; many of them had chopped wood the day before and had sore backs. They didn't understand chiropractic, just like most people – but this isn't their fault. It's the profession's fault for not explaining what chiropractic care really is.

My purpose in this chapter is to help you understand why chiropractic care makes up one of the four pillars of true health and well-being. After finishing this chapter my hope is that you will understand that chiropractic care isn't a drug-free way to alleviate pain but a lifestyle choice that makes sense as a preventative measure, just like eating nutrient dense food, staying active, and talking to yourself in a natural manner (I will be talking about this in a later chapter).

B. J. Palmer, the son of the founder of chiropractic, said it well:

> "In the future, chiropractic will be valued for its preventative qualities as much as for relieving and adjusting the cause of ailments."

As a chiropractor, I treat patients by restoring normal motion and alignment in spinal joints. Whether or not this makes a disease go away is not important. Normal spinal motion is necessary for proper brain and nervous system function. This has a positive effect on the human body as a whole.

Our spine is the most neglected organ – just ask someone who has suffered from acute low back pain. They are not able to do anything! Not only is it completely debilitating, it is also the number one reason people miss time from work. I once read a statement that went something like this: Have you ever heard of a spine transplant? I haven't. You only get one, so take care of it.

Our nervous system primarily does four things. It controls every movement we make. It is involved in everything we sense or feel. Nerves also control and regulate every body function, from digestion to circulation to respiration to reproduction. The nervous system also allows us to relate to the outside world.

As we begin to understand the importance of our spine and nervous system, we begin to appreciate it more and more, and more importantly find the desire take care of it.

Chiropractic care is only used by about 10 percent of the U.S. population. Most people have no idea what I do as a chiropractor. In this chapter, you will not only learn about one of the pillars of true health and wellness, but you will learn a lot of new terminology that I hope you will begin to use as you talk about health and wellness with your loved ones.

The first term I want to explain is a lesion I actually treat as a chiropractor – the subluxation. The subluxation, in medical terms, is just a partial dislocation, however in chiropractic it involves much more, which you will learn throughout this chapter. In chiropractic, physically it is a slight misalignment of the vertebra one to another or the first vertebrae of the neck to the base of the skull or the last vertebra in the low back to the sacrum. This can be a misalignment that is either dynamic (with movement) or static (without movement).

What causes this misalignment in the spine? Or, in other words, why should I involve chiropractic care in my wellness lifestyle? Three reasons: toxins, thoughts, and traumas. The founder of chiropractic, D.D. Palmer, called these the Three T's. Today, science, along with the studies by Hans Selye about stress, back up much of what D.D. Palmer said more than a hundred years ago.

I am certain that each and every one of us have one of these Three T's in our life at this moment, and many of us have had them for years even decades.

The First T – Toxins.

Toxins are environmental stressors. They're all around us, and we face more of them every day. People living in cities are exposed to more than 70,000 toxins daily! When we think of toxins we think of something physical entering our body. There are many different types of toxins. As it is now, more people in the world live in cities than not. The city is a very unnatural place to live. We as humans were never meant to live on top of each other in high-rise buildings. In cities we not only find physical toxins but toxicity in noise stimulation and in visual stimulation. Modern society practically lives in front of a screen, be it a smart phone, tablet, computer, or television screen. This can be decreased dramatically with changes in lifestyle, like having a certain time of day when all electronics are turned off and taking time to regularly leave the city and enjoy nature, really return to our roots. In one of my podcast episodes(1) I interviewed Elijah Szasz. For twenty-one days, he lived with a machine that read all the different types of radiation he received from cell phone waves, internet waves, and other waves that surrounded him. It is amazing the amount of these waves we receive daily.

Not only are we over stimulated in the city, we are also bombarded with physical toxins like vehicle contamination, industrial contamination, cigarette smoke, and contaminants that we find in new houses and buildings. I've read that over 10,000 chemicals are used in the construction and maintenance of new homes. However, probably the two worst toxins of our modern society are prescribed medication and our modern food system.

The pharmaceutical companies make billions of dollars by keeping the people sick. Their job is not to cure people – that would put them out of work. Their job is to keep you on a medication for as long as possible. Our bodies are never deficient in prescribed medication, that I can promise you. However, we see more and more medication that is used as a lifestyle. You don't take it to get over a serious crisis – you take it for the rest of your life! In the United States the number of people taking a prescribed medication has reached almost 60 percent. In other words, three in five people are talking a prescribed medication that will probably be taken for the rest of their lives, unless they make the appropriate changes in their lifestyle.

Not only do we see a huge increase in the amount of prescribed medication being taken in the properly diagnosed amount, we also see a huge increase in the abuse of prescription drugs. More than 15 million people in the United States abuse prescription drugs. That number is higher than the combined abuse of cocaine, hallucinogens, inhalers, and heroin. Depressants, opioids, and antidepressants are responsible for more overdose deaths than cocaine, heroin, methamphetamine and amphetamines combined. Almost 50 percent of teens believe that prescription drugs are much safer than illegal street drugs. Between 60 and 70 percent say that home medicine cabinets are their source of drugs. Pharmaceutical drugs are even found in the public water supply of many places due to the amount of drugs being discarded through drains. Even those not taking a pharmaceutical drug are being affected by this toxin. This is probably one of the hardest things for people to understand. We have been raised for generations now thinking that pills are what cure us. We couldn't be further from the truth. Yes, a pill can decrease a symptom, but it will never cure anything. We must understand that we need to work very hard to eliminate the amount of drugs we are allowing into our ecosystem of cells.

Before I continue, I must explain that modern medicine has its role in health. Many reading may think that I am completely against modern medicine. No, modern medicine has its role in health and it is a very important role. Modern medicine has achieved what we can call miracles in crisis care. The lives modern medicine has saved in emergency situations is mind blowing. I personally have experienced the effects of modern medicine in my own life, and thanks to modern medicine my son is with me today. However, we must understand the role of modern medicine because if we look at the overall health of the people, it has consistently decreased over the years. Every year we see more and more sick people, and at the same time we see more doctors, more nurses, more hospitals, more surgeries, and more medication.

The role of modern medicine is for emergencies and should only be used for emergencies. Emergencies are usually short moments in life. A pill, if going to be taken, should be taken in emergencies only, and only for a very short while with a clear plan to stop as soon as possible. On the other hand, the job of wellness practitioners is to help in the maintenance of our health and well-being. This is a constant and ongoing process that is lifelong. Our goal should be to use modern medicine as little as possible and visit wellness practitioners often to help in the maintenance of a healthy ecosystem. We should never wait until our health is at a crisis. Emergencies happen, and we have a wonderful system that can save lives during emergencies and crisis. However, let's live a lifestyle of wellness so we can avoid all the pain, suffering, and heartache that many preventable emergencies bring.

The other major toxicity in our daily lives is our food system. I talked extensively about this in the chapter about nutrient dense food. We avoid some of the worst toxins there are – pesticides, herbicides, fungicides, and chemical fertilizers – when we make sure we are eating properly raised food. The effects of these toxins on our ecosystem of cells are becoming more and more understood as time goes by. We must avoid at all cost foods laced with these chemicals!

The Second T – Thoughts.

In other words, this is the way we talk to ourselves, the way we see ourselves in the mirror, the way we treat ourselves. Unhealthy self talk is pandemic. We see images on all the screens we can't get away from and long to be like these images. That can mean either physically or socially. Modern society tries to portray certain beliefs, certain looks, and certain ways of portraying yourself, trying to fit us all into a specific image or way of life. Again, this could not be further from the truth. We are all very unique in our own special ways, and that is what makes the world such a beautiful place and a great place to live in. This is the main reason I continue to work personally with patients. I love how everybody is completely unique. Every person returns to health and wellness in their unique way. Of course there are four pillars that we must be concerned about as we build the lifestyle to truly be well, however each person reacts and reaches this unique lifestyle in their own way.

We need to return to our natural way of seeing ourselves. We are born happy, and as we learn to communicate, we communicate happiness not just to ourselves but to those around us. Those with little ones or those that had little ones around once can testify to this. Little kids are naturally happy. This does not mean they don't have their times of sadness, however the ability to forgive and forget is probably one of the best examples us as adults could learn from.

The Third T – Traumas.

This deals with two types of traumas: macro traumas and micro traumas. Most people who go to a chiropractor are there because of some type of a macro trauma, like a motor vehicle crash or a sports injury. Most macro traumas are rare, and many people may never even experience a macro trauma in their lifetime. Micro traumas are completely different. None of us are exempt from experiencing micro traumas. The micro traumas of life are the repetitive motions, also known as overuse injuries, the chronic bad posture we see in schools, workplaces, and homes, and the chronic sedentary lifestyles we see more and more of and at younger and younger ages. We have become a society that lives our lives in the sitting position. Even worse than that, we then have our heads tilted forward looking into either a computer screen, iPad or iPhone. We truly could not put our spines into a worse position. This happens day in and day out and is starting at a younger age every year!

These traumas, which we can also call accidents and injuries to our tissues, actually tear tissues that hold the spine together. This includes muscles, tendons, ligaments, and joint capsules. We can also see changes on the bony surfaces of the joints. This creates a weakness, which allows the spine to break down, causing it to lock into a distressed position. This changes how the body functions and results in decreased motion in joints and the tissues that surround them. As a result, we see muscle tension. Our physiology also changes, and all this happens subconsciously. For example, we see an increase in nociception and a decrease in proprioception.

These are two words that should be common knowledge for all people who live a lifestyle of wellness. Nociception comes from the Latin word *nocere,* which means to harm or hurt. Nociceptors are found throughout the body, from our skin to organs. Nociceptors are the body's response to noxious stimuli, or in other words stressors. They can be chemical, mechanical, or thermal. When our joints are in the distressed position for long periods of time we see an increase in overall nociception stimulation due to the mechanical stressor of the distressed joint. All this happens while we are not feeling a single physical symptom.

It is incredible the amount of times I have cared for new patients who have come to the clinic with excruciating low back pain for the first time in their lives. Many times for reasons that should never cause such intense pain. I take radiographs of their spine and find degeneration of the joints of the spine. The decades of the joint locked into the distressed position caused the spine to degenerate, all while the patient did not even know it was happening.

Nociception, the body's response to stressors, triggers the activities of the stress response. This is what makes the lesion I treat as a chiropractor so important! The joints in the distressed position not only cause an increase in the degeneration of the joint, it also activates the stress response. Who has not heard about all the ill effects of a chronic stress response? Most people leave the doctor's office with instructions to decrease stress as a primary way to improve health.

To fully understand why chiropractic is one of the four pillars to health and true well-being we must understand the ill effects of the stress response.

The stress response – why chiropractic is one of the four pillars to true health.

The lesion I treat, the subluxation, as a stressor to the body, triggers the stress response which activates the sympathetic nervous system. Once activated, we start to see many changes in our physiology, the way our body is functioning.

We see an increase in the stress hormones that have become more well known lately. The sympathetic nervous system sends signals directly to the adrenal glands that sit just above the kidneys where the stress hormones are secreted, which include cortisol, and the catecholamines that consist of epinephrine, norepinephrine, adrenaline, and noradrenaline.

Catecholamines cause many changes in how our body functions. First, we will see an increase in heart rate and vasoconstriction of the arteries, which is simply the narrowing of the arteries. This is done to increase blood flow because the body needs the stress hormones and the energy to deal with the stressor now! One change we will see during stress is an increase in blood pressure, this being intelligent during the stressful moment, which should be short lived.

The catecholamines also cause the freeing of fatty acids that are then used to make more energy. We also see cortisol breaking down the protein stored and working on the liver, causing the breakdown of the glycogen stores also to make more energy that is so needed during the stress response. Catecholamines and cortisol also decrease the amount of insulin receptors there are on the cell wall, which will cause an increase in the amount of of blood sugar. This causes an increase in blood insulin levels. Insulin, when chronically found in the blood, is now known to also trigger the stress response, increase the amount of calcium found in urine, decrease the amount of insulin-like growth factor, and lower magnesium levels.

Why does the body begin to break down protein for energy? Why does it break down glycogen stores for increased energy? Why does it free up fatty acids to be able to make more energy substrate? The stress response, when activated under normal circumstances, needs to provide a lot of energy to get us out of danger's way or help us fight our way out or survive a period of scarcity. That is why the stress response is also known as the "fight or flight response."

We not only convert protein and fatty acids to energy substrate and break down our glycogen stores, but our bodies also begin to crave the substances that are needed to produce the energy necessary to support the stress response, which are sugars and fats!

Cortisol also acts on cholesterol levels. Similar to how it reduces the amount of insulin receptors there are on the cell wall, it also reduces the amount of insulin receptors for low density lipoprotein, which is LDL cholesterol. This means the cells will be taking in a lot less cholesterol, which is smart. The possibility of getting hurt during the acute stress response is very high and cholesterol is used in healing cuts or lesions. Cholesterol is also used in the building of the stress hormones.

While we are on the topic, cholesterol is also very important in cell membrane health. The cell membrane is what protects each cell. It is the gate where everything must check in first before entering. Without a healthy cell membrane the cell has no chance of survival. It also is what gives the cell its shape and what helps it connect to other cells to form tissue. Let's stop blaming cholesterol for so many diseases and get to the base of it all. We all know deep down that the real problems are our lifestyle choices!

The stress response also causes an increase in the clotting factors, like plasmin in the blood. It does this to be ready for any possible trauma that can, and usually will, occur during an acute stress response.

All these changes occur while stressed. These are changes that we see throughout the body, but what about all the changes we see mentally? There are just as many changes mentally as there are physically when we are stressed.

The stress response works on various parts of the brain to help us survive a stressful environment. The stress response is not only to help us survive, it is also used to remind ourselves to never put ourselves in that stressful environment again.

All this happens in various places in the brain like the amygdala, which deals with the processing of memory, decision making, and emotional reactions. When we are stressed, our emotional or anxious memories dominate. This is so we don't put ourselves in that same environment again.

Catecholamines also work on the hippocampus, where we see a suppression of working memory. Working memory is responsible for the temporary holding, processing, and use of information. Working memory is an important process for reasoning and the guidance of decision making and behavior. It also suppresses the ability to focus our attention and the learning of facts. This also intelligent, because when we are in a situation of survival there is no immediate need to focus and learn something new.

During the stress response we also see the activation of the locus coeruleus, which is the principal site of the brain for the synthesis of noradrenaline. Noradrenaline affects our sleep-wake cycle, attention and memory, cognitive control, emotions, posture, and balance. When noradrenaline is produced and released, it acts on certain areas of the brain, which cause the suppression of our short term memory and rational behavior and the activation of the areas of the brain that deal with emotional learning and instinctual behavior.

Not only that, but noradrenaline during the stress response causes our sensory systems to become even more sharp in their perception of stimuli. The sensory systems affected include vision, hearing, touch, taste, smell, balance, and movement. In a chronically stressed person the slightest touch can cause discomfort. Michael Meaney, Ph.D. put it best when he said,

> "stress sharpens the signal detection system at the cost of concentration."

Due to the increased release of noradrenaline, a person that is under a lot of stress becomes easily distracted.

We are not done yet. Noradrenaline released from the locus coeruleus is inhibited by a chemical called serotonin. Serotonin is known as one of the major mood neurotransmitters in our brains. When serotonin levels are low, we're more depressed, and when they're high, we're happier. Well, when we are chronically stressed the creation of serotonin cannot keep up with the creation of noradrenaline, and fatigue causes a drop in serotonin levels, causing a drop in our mood.

Chronic stress is involved in pretty much every modern metabolic disease we see today, from diabetes to cancer. Stress reduction is one of the most important ways to improve our health and well-being, whether we are symptom free or not.

Toxins, thoughts, and traumas are stressors. Our bodies react to these stressors in intelligent ways, however in today's lifestyle we encounter these different types of stress on a constant basis forcing our bodies to be stressed chronically.

You might be saying yes, I understand how traumas can cause this stress to the joint and activate the stress response, but how do the other two involve the lesion I treat, the subluxation? It all comes back to the stress response and how we as humans work as holistic beings. We need to look at ourselves as an ecosystem of cells that work harmoniously together.

Health cannot be compartmentalized. Thoughts stress us emotionally. Chronic emotional stressors, like all chronic stressors, lead to chronic muscle tension. This tension causes spasms, metabolic changes, and other problems. This chronic tension then causes, or worsens, the distressed joint of the spine. Toxins do the very same. This works both ways. The distressed joint causes an increase in the stress response, causing muscle tension, metabolic changes, and other problems making us more susceptible to the emotional and toxic stressors we find in our daily lives. The Three T's work simultaneously with each other and must be treated as one. That is why we cannot only treat our patients with chiropractic adjustments. We must involve coaching on what is consumed, the amount of movement is achieved, and how close one is to speaking and seeing themselves in a natural manner. Chronic stress, no matter where it comes from, continually activates our sympathetic nervous system, which causes all the physiological changes of the stress response in our bodies.

Eustress—the other side of stress

While we are on the subject, I want to talk a little about the importance of stress in our lives. Yup, you heard that right—we also need stress in our lives. Not just any stress, but acute stress. Episodes of short-lived stress are fundamental in our health and well-being.

Eustress is a beneficial stress. The term was coined by endocrinologist Hans Selye, and it consists of the Greek prefix eu- meaning "good," and stress, literally meaning "good stress." It really comes down to how we perceive the stressful event. It is the positive response to stress. This response is healthy; it gives a feeling of fulfillment or other positive feelings.

If you think that all stress is harmful and that we must rid ourselves of it completely, you are leaving out an important part of our development as humans.

When we look at the stress response in acute situations we must understand that it is not harmful at all. The stress response is always the most intelligent path our bodies can take in that moment; it is getting us ready for whatever might happen next. Our ancestors usually had to run from a predator, fight their way out of a dangerous situation, or endure various days without food. Nowadays that stressful situation might be you on the foul line, down by one with no time left on the clock and two foul shots to win the championship game. Or perhaps you're in front of a crowd about to give your first, or fiftieth, talk. It could even be you waiting in my waiting room, about to be treated with chiropractic care for the first time.

What happens with your physiology when you go through one of the above situations? First, your heart rate is going to go up. You might also start to sweat. Most people will think this is bad, that we are anxious or not coping well, when really, this is all good and normal. You are actually coping well to the situation.

We must change our outlook of these changes in our physiology. Don't think that you are doing things wrong if you feel anxious or worried or stressed out. Literally, this is your body being intelligent. We need to see our stress response as helpful in these types of situations. The next time your heart is pounding from stress, think to yourself, "This is my body helping me rise to this challenge."

When you understand stress in this way, your stress response becomes healthier. It is now known that when you view the stress response as helpful, your heart will still pound just as fast and just as hard, but your blood vessels will stay relaxed. When you view the stress response as helpful, it actually changes physiology to the same physiology of when we have moments of joy and courage.

I have talked about catecholamines and cortisol as stress hormones, but there are other stress hormones that we don't hear about as often. One is oxytocin. One of oxytocin's functions is to sharpen the brain's social instincts. It motivates you to do things that improve relationships.

Why would the body increase the amount of oxytocin during a stressful event?

When you are stressed, your body is trying to motivate you to seek support. Your stress response is telling you to tell someone how you feel, instead of bottling it up. Your stress response also wants to make sure you notice when others in your life are struggling so that you can support them. When life becomes difficult, your stress response wants you to be surrounded by people who care about you.

The body could not be anymore intelligent. It knows exactly what it needs to heal and to stay healthy. As an animal species that thrives in communities and not alone, you do the one thing that you most need when you are down and stressed out—you secrete a hormone that makes you want to receive help or be of help to others. It helps you open up and improves your relationships.

Oxytocin also acts on the body, helping heart cells regenerate and heal from any stress-induced damage. This stress hormone strengthens your heart.

When the body is stressed, it knows that it needs to increase blood pressure and pump the energy substrate and stress hormone faster in order to get it to where it is needed as fast as possible. To counteract this change that should be short lived, it increases another hormone to help heal the muscle that had to work so hard to save us from the stressful situation. It is also a natural anti-inflammatory and it helps your blood vessels stay relaxed during stress.

To truly be healthy and well, you must activate the stress response. It's important to understand that stress needs to be something that is short lived. Those short moments in life like that shot from the foul line or that 45-minute presentation in front of a crowd or waiting for your first chiropractic treatment in my waiting room can be a benefit to you and your body. Your body is beyond intelligent, something none of us will ever fully understand. Stress is the most intelligent decision our body makes in the environments we put it in. Deep inside, it is telling us we have what it takes to battle this challenge. Never forget this. Believe in yourself, and believe in your natural self.

Now, back to the importance of chiropractic care in your wellness lifestyle. There are two types of movement in the nervous system. Efferent movement is the movement of nerve impulses coming from inside the brain, moving outward, while afferent movement is the movement of nerve impulses coming inside the brain from outside receptors. This is how we experience everything around us. The amount of information that gets sent to the brain is extraordinarily more than what actually leaves the brain. I have read numbers of up to 3 trillion bits of information get sent to the brain every second, however only 50 bits of that information actually gets to the conscious part of the brain. In other words, only 50 bits of information gets sent out.

Afferent movement is very important. Much of the information that gets sent to the brain is through proprioceptors. This is the other term that should become common use when we talk about true health and wellness. Proprioception comes from the Latin word proprius, meaning "one's own" or "individual" and capio or capere, which means "to take" or "grasp." Proprioception is the sense of the relative position of neighboring parts of the body and strength of effort being employed in movement. Basically, proprioceptors let us know where we are in space, blindfolded or not.

Go ahead and try this. Lift one of your arms up. Of course, you know your arm is raised because you can see it. Now, close your eyes and lift up that same arm. You knew your arm was raised because of proprioception.

When we have distressed joints, the amount of proprioception input that gets to the brain is reduced. This is important because proprioceptors have such a vital role in the proper function of the cerebellum. The cerebellum was known for many years as the place where fine movement is achieved. We do not make choppy movement because of the cerebellum. However, it is now known that the cerebellum not only makes our movements sharp and clear, but it also sharpens our balance and coordination, cognition, learning, emotion, and the function of our organs, including the immune organs. This is huge – the effect of the distressed joint deals with practically every physiological process of the body.

Proprioceptors also help in the suppression of nociception getting to the brain. Remember that nociception is our brain's detection of noxious stimuli and stressors. When our body receives too much nociceptive input, the stress response is activated and we see all the physiological effects of that. And when chronic, it causes havoc on our ecosystem of cells, which will eventually cause disease. The majority of this happens without us even knowing. It happens all subconsciously. These metabolic diseases like diabetes, heart disease, autoimmune diseases, and cancers don't happen overnight. They take many years of chronic stress response activation, usually decades.

This is why chiropractic must be part of our wellness lifestyle. Unless we experience some type of macro trauma it can be decades before we actually feel a physical symptom like pain from a distressed joint. Worst of all, we will have decades of an activated stress response causing havoc on our body's physiology, or in other words, the way our body is functioning. Chiropractic is so much more than pain relief. Doctor of Chiropractic Christopher Kent stated it perfectly when he said,

> "Although stimulation of articular mechanoreceptors may exert an analgesic effect, use of manipulation for the episodic, symptomatic treatment of pain is not chiropractic."

This is why my great-grandfather went to a small Iowa town in the 1920's to become a chiropractor. Four generations later, I went to the same small town and became a chiropractor – for the very same reasons.

(1) pastosverdesfarm.libsyn.com/21-day-challenge-with-elijah-szasz-062

Natural internal dialogue
Exactly that – natural!

To be healthy and well we must understand the impacts of our thoughts, our internal dialogue on our health.

Negative self-talk is a stressor. That is the key! When we talk to ourselves in a way that is not natural we are intoxicating our ecosystem of cells. It has the same effect on our physiology as any toxin, from chemicals in our food that is ingested to the breathing of vehicle contamination. Negative self-talk is a toxin! If we see it as it really is – a toxin – we can more fully understand the importance of avoiding it at all costs. Imagine each negative thought as a person in a white rubber suit with yellow gloves and a gas mask, spraying the fields with a pesticide. Would you even go close to that field? No! That is exactly how we must treat negative self-talk; we must stay as far away as possible.

Unnatural internal dialogue as a stressor will activate the sympathetic nervous system, which in turn activates the stress response causing an increase in the stress hormones, cortisol and the catecholamines. These activate certain parts of the brain: the amygdala, which deals with emotion; the hippocampus, which deals with learning and concentration; and the hypothalamus, which deals with sleep and emotional activity. With the activation of the stress response the body's physiology changes. When this physiology becomes chronic, we begin to see many of the health problems present in modern society.

What I have seen over and over again in clinical practice as I take a history of a patient is how often they go through life without any major physical trauma, but how, after a major emotional event, like the passing of a loved one or divorce, they suddenly begin to experience some type of physical symptom, the number one being pain. Usually, the pain is in the lower neck and mid to upper back. They don't understand how to cope with the loss and become depressed, causing negative self-talk. This mental state eventually causes a physical symptom. In other words, we function in a holistic manner. Everything works together. We cannot separate the physical from the mental or the spiritual. You can have mental pain or pain that is even deeper, spiritual pain and experience it in a physical manner.

An important component of self-talk is that we have total control. I know, many times it feels like we don't, but the truth is that we have total control of what we say to ourselves. We don't have control of what may happen around us, but the way we react to our environment is completely under our control. I don't think there is a better example of just this than Victor Frankl. His book, Man's Search for Meaning, is an account of his life in a Nazi concentration camp and how his experiences solidified what he had taught as a psychologist. He stated that,

> "Forces beyond your control can take away everything you possess except one thing, your freedom to choose how you will respond to the situation. You cannot control what happens to you in life, but you can always control what you will feel and do about what happens to you."

There may be times when you feel that there is no hope, that there is no way you can change how you talk to yourself or see yourself in the mirror. We can get to a point of feeling like this because of something called neuroplasticity. Our neurons work like a stream of water. The stream of water always looks for the easiest route; the more water that goes through the same route the easier it becomes. When we use negative self-talk we are forming a neural pathway; every time we use that pathway it becomes more and more sensitized. It becomes easier to use the pathway of negative self-talk because it becomes the pathway of least resistance. That is why once you are on the path it seems harder and harder to overcome. However, the opposite happens when we constantly think positive thoughts. The positive thought pathways also become sensitized and it becomes easier and easier to have positive self-talk. Either way, it is a journey and one that takes time and effort.

We need to look at our mental strength as our physical strength; we don't build muscle over night. It is a process of constantly working and building. Our mental strength comes in the exact same manner, so we must work hard to build our mental strength. This hard work is very satisfying. What makes living the wellness lifestyle so wonderful is once we are strong physically and mentally the maintenance is also extremely satisfying. And it only gets easier and easier because of neuroplasticity!

The more we talk to ourselves in a positive manner – or really, the more we talk to ourselves in a natural way – the easier it becomes! There are many great examples out there to follow, but as I go through life and see my own children and the children around me, I see more and more how children live a lifestyle of wellness and don't even know it. In so many ways they are being a great example to us adults. They still have the natural lifestyle in them; they live, or at least try to live, how all humans should. It is us, as adults, who get in the way. Children still want to jump in the mud, they still want to play in the dirt, they still sit and move in a natural manner, and they constantly have a smile on their faces. They are incredibly fast to forgive and forget, and possess a love that is unconditional. Many people use the word 'innate' when they talk about our natural characteristics. I have learned over time that 'natural' is easier to understand. They act how we adults should be acting naturally.

The other day, we had one of our three-year-old nieces over to stay the night. She sat on one of the stairs leading to the second floor, and for the whole time she sat straight, with the natural curve in her low back and her chin tucked in. It was amazing to see her do this and not feel uncomfortable in any way. This wasn't for a couple of seconds, either, but for a prolonged period of time. Just like how we lose our natural manner of movement and posture over time, we also seem to lose that natural way of talking to ourselves. We forget those natural belief systems we are born with that allow us to reach our potential.

It saddens me how we let life knock us down over and over again, until we slowly forget who we truly are. We are beings with an incredible ability to self-heal and to self-regulate. We have an enormous potential to create and to build. We are all naturally good and look to help. These are not traits that need to be learned – we are born with them. I am more and more convinced that each and every one of us, no matter where we are from or our current condition in life, all have the ability both mentally and physically to do great things in life.

While talking with my mother-in-law the other day, she brought up a medical doctor she had read about in an article that was going through a very difficult challenge in life. We will all have our challenges in life, our learning experiences. The way this person became a medical doctor really impressed me. This man, as a boy, came from a very poor family from Paraguay who decided that his purpose and meaning in life was to help people feel better. He didn't have the money to go to a medical school, so he left Paraguay and went to Argentina alone where education was a lot more economical. During his studies, he lived in the poorest conditions imaginable. But he persevered until he received his medical degree. As a medical doctor, he focused his efforts in helping those who lived in the same conditions he had lived in for so many years. This boy, who turned into a man, demonstrated and retained what we all have naturally – the will to be good and do good, even in the poorest conditions. We all have this same natural ability to build what we want in life.

There are many ways to help us return to talking to ourselves in a natural way, and I have found a morning routine is a great way to start.

The morning routine – a great start!

Every day, I start my morning by doing certain things. First, get up and drink a glass of water. I do this to get my digestive juices rolling. I then make my bed. I don't do it because I love to make beds; I did enough bed making in the Marine Corps for a lifetime. I still remember that 45-degree flip of the blanket I had to have perfect when I tucked in my sheets and blanket. I make my bed because it's a great way to start my day off with an easy accomplishment. I can have the worst day and be just hanging on by a thread, but know I accomplished something: I got up and made the bed. It's also nice to come home to a nicely made bed after a tough day.

Second, I drink a tea called yerba mate. My wife and I enjoy this custom because we're both of Argentine descent. We talk about the upcoming day and what we want to accomplish while drinking mate together. The third thing I do, not in any particular order mind you, is take a couple of minutes to pray, meditate, and clear my mind. My fourth habit is to write in my journal.

I start my days off by doing at least three of these four things. If I don't do one of them for some odd reason, I don't kick myself – I just keep "crushing it." These are the exact words I write in my journal. Almost every morning, I get my journal out, set the timer on my phone for five minutes, and I write what I need to get done that day, what I'm thankful for, and how I'm going to act that day. But, before I write all that, I write, "TODAY I AM GOING TO CRUSH IT!!!"

The morning routine is very important, it is the time we have to reflect on how we will use one of the most precious gifts we have – time! Each day we start fresh. It doesn't matter how the day before went; we get a fresh start. The morning routine helps us build the mindset we need to take on another day with the right attitude. It also helps us as we tackle our daily activities. We will all have different morning routines. Mine has these four components. I recommend you use at least two, journaling and meditation, every morning and then add whatever you believe makes a great morning routine.

The morning routine also helps to constantly remind us of our purpose, or our meaning in life. Why you are here! Much of the negative self-talk begins when we forget our purpose in life, or when we begin to think there is no meaning in life. We all have our own special meaning in life. With a morning routine and the daily reminder of who you are and what your goals are, what your plan is, you can stay focused on the important aspects of life. These will all be different for each and every one of us, however I can promise you that checking Facebook or Instagram is not it! I also know that becoming wealthy is not your meaning to life, nor is it your purpose. When you find your true meaning the rest will come. The more we look to become wealthy, the more we will miss it. We shouldn't seek wealth; only if we work towards our true meaning to this life will true wealth be found. With patience wealth just happens in time as we find our meaning in life and pursue it.

As a whole, the morning routine helps prevent a lot of stress that we would otherwise experience. It's a great start in helping us organize and prepare not only our thoughts but also our actions for the day. As we become more organized with our time we find time for the most important things in life. I love Ernest C. Wilson's look at time. He said,

> "We deceive ourselves when we say we have not time. Every one has the same amount of time - all the time there is."

We can accomplish everything, but it comes down to how we plan and use our time.

We have now learned that stress – it doesn't matter what type of stress, be it mental, physical, or spiritual – causes certain changes in how we function. Our bodies react to stress in the same way, as well as when we ponder on past stressful events or worry about events in the future that might be stressful. I have found a lifestyle choice that helps prevent a lot of the worrying about future events that may happen. I recommend it as one of the many choices you can make as you begin or continue your journey through life living a lifestyle of wellness.

Modern survivalism and the wellness lifestyle.

How can I decrease my overall stress?

That's a very good question!

One of the best answers is just to simplify your life. We live in a world that makes everything too complex. I've read articles from people three times my age who've recognized certain patterns in life. They've experienced good and bad times, ups and downs, periods of joy and sadness, and cycles of plenty and scarcity. When our lives turn in unanticipated and undesirable directions, we often experience stress and anxiety. We must face the challenge of not allowing life's stresses and strains to get the better of us. We must endure the various seasons of life while remaining positive – and even optimistic!

Henry David Thoreau was an author, poet, philosopher, abolitionist, naturalist, tax resister, development critic, surveyor, and historian. However, he is best known for his book Walden, a reflection upon simple living in natural surroundings, and his essay "Civil Disobedience," an argument for disobeying unjust states.

In March 1845, Thoreau separated himself from the world for a while to simplify his life and figure out what it's all about. In Walden, he explained how he settled on a piece of property owned by his good friend, Ralph Waldo Emerson, at a place called Walden Pond. He purchased a small, crudely built shack from a railroad worker and tore it down. He constructed a cabin from these materials and lumber from the woods. He kept financial records of his efforts and concluded he spent $28.12 for a home and freedom. He planted a garden of peas, potatoes, corn, beans, and turnips to sustain his simple life. He planted two-and-a-half acres of beans with the intent of using these small profits to cover his needs – he earned $8.71.

In his cabin, Thoreau lived quite independent of time. He had neither a clock nor a calendar. He spent his time writing and studying the beauties and wonders of nature that surrounded him – including local plants, birds, and animals. However, he didn't live the life of a hermit. He visited the town of Concord most days and invited friends to his cabin for conversations. When two years had passed, he left his cabin behind without regret. He considered his time there the proper amount to accomplish his purpose: to experience the benefits of a simplified lifestyle. From his experiences at Walden Pond, Thoreau determined a man needs only four things: food, clothing, shelter, and fuel. I'm not saying we need to simplify our lives to that extent, but we should simplify our lifestyles.

Another great way to decrease your overall stress is to prepare for what life throws at you. The tenets of modern survivalism can help enormously; they're an important part of a healthy lifestyle. You may or may not be well prepared for the challenges life can throw at you. However, your level of preparedness isn't important – what matters is getting started and moving ahead one step at a time.

I returned to my roots. I say this because all of us, at one point, were modern survivalists (or, at least, our ancestors were). A couple of months before the start of the 2008 economic crisis in the United States, I was in my second trimester at Palmer College of Chiropractic. I remember talking with another student about the situation in the country.

My friend and I talked about politics and how nothing ever changes; it doesn't matter whether a Republican or a Democrat is in office. We talked about preparing for a dollar collapse (which could certainly happen). He brought up an interesting novel by James Wesley Rawles called Patriots. This book wasn't just a novel; it offered a lot of practical knowledge. He lent me his copy, which I read in four days. This was a pretty fast pace, considering I was taking about fifty credit hours of classes at that time.

At this point, I started returning to my roots; I started thinking about preparedness again. I had been brought up with a preparedness mindset; I just wasn't putting it into practice at that time. I grew up in a small southern Utah town; we had a huge garden, chickens, goats, pigs, and a horse. Most of the food I ate came from our garden or our animals. However, my family's lifestyle changed when we moved to Las Vegas, NV. I know – this is probably one of the worst places I could have lived, a populated desert. In Las Vegas, my parents tried to grow a garden. However, it was quite difficult; their yields were very small.

I still remember when the housing bubble finally popped. I was at college; all of a sudden, I had to change the lenders for my student loans. Many students were scared and thought they wouldn't be able to get new loans for the next trimester. Were they ever wrong! We continued to get loans, and our tuition increased every trimester. It's hard to believe how much my "piece of paper" cost me.

As a side note, people who say a college education is the only way to go have no idea. Debt is cancer; avoid it at all costs.

Now, back to how it all began. After reading the book Patriots, I read articles every day on survivalblog.com (while also studying other things). I learned about 72-hour kits and bug-out bags and even created my own bug-out bag. I'm still in the process six years later, and am always updating it. My wife and I started storing food and planted our first garden. Though we were poor students, we saved a couple ounces of silver. As my survivalism philosophy developed, I discovered modern survivalism and its tenets, which changed the way I thought about survivalism.

At its core, modern survivalism involves preparing for and avoiding (or at least limiting) life's most stressful moments. Chronic stress reduces our overall health. These stressful moments can be personal (like a job loss) or general (like a pandemic). To deal with stressful incidents, we have to live "in the now" and avoid thinking about the past or the future. It's very important to understand our situations and our circles of influence. We must understand what we can personally do to improve our situations and not concern ourselves with things we can't change. Awakening to our situations generally happens in five stages: denial, anger, bargaining, depression, and finally, acceptance.

Once we accept our situations, another important part of modern survivalism is using our mental, physical, and financial resources to better our lives today. We should prepare for all potential crises by considering our five basic human needs: water, food, shelter, defense, and hygiene/health. An attractive aspect of modern survivalism is that if a crisis never materializes, we're better off for having prepared.

I learned the term 'modern survivalism' from a gentleman named Jack Spirko, a modern survivalist who lives in Texas. As an entrepreneur, Jack Spirko started "The Survival Podcast;" I started listening to this show in 2008 and highly recommend it. I'm grateful for Jack's work in the world of modern survivalism. I also learned a great deal from a gentleman named Fernando Aguirre. Fernando, an Argentine, lived through his country's 2001 economic crisis. He blogs and vlogs about his experiences in this crisis (and what he learned after) at www.ferfal.blogspot.com. He's written two books, which I also recommend. Fernando left Argentina, lived in

Northern Ireland for a couple of years, and now resides in Spain.

A couple of Jack Spirko's tenets explain modern survivalism very well. I'll use them as my basis for explaining the modern survivalism lifestyle. Please visit his website at www.thesurvivalpodcast.com and read his tenets of modern survivalism. I'm not an expert in modern survivalism, but, like many people, I learn more every day.

Modern survivalists employ a variety of principles. The most important one is, as Jack says,

> "Everything you do should improve your position in life even if nothing goes wrong."

Modern survivalists are realists who know things sometimes go wrong, and it's better to be prepared than to expect others to solve your problems. This is the core of his philosophy (and mine, as well). Prepared and self-sufficient lifestyles reduce our overall stress. Blend all of your preparations into your lifestyle, so they improve your life situation – even if disaster never strikes.

There are many ways to prepare for stressful situations.

First, grow your own food. Vegetable gardening is for everyone, whether you have a balcony garden or a 1000-acre farm. Once you eat something you've grown, there's no going back!

Gardens can help you provide for your family in stressful times; they also improve your physical health by providing necessary nutrients. And, if that wasn't enough, they also improve your emotional health. Scientists have shown that working in fertile soil physiologically improves our mental health. This is accomplished by a bacterium called mycobacterium vaccae, which is found only in rich soil. It triggers serotonin, which elevates our moods, decreases our anxiety, and improves our cognitive functions.

Producing some of your own food is a very important part of stress reduction. Food storage is an exceptional investment. Food is one of the most important things to have in a crisis. For example, if you lost your job, you'd be glad to know you didn't have to worry about food because it's stored in your pantry and waiting in your garden. You could focus solely on finding a new income source. I recommend starting your own business if you're looking for a new job.

Second, debt is financial cancer. Pay off your debt as soon as possible and avoid it at all costs. Debt causes enormous stress. I should know – I went to Palmer College of Chiropractic and accumulated way too much debt for the "piece of paper" I was given. In every way possible, debt changes the ways we make economic decisions. It's been a weight on my shoulders and has, at certain times in the last few years, had me on my knees in despair.

Third, modern survivalism is important to the wellness lifestyle because it helps you prioritize things. Plan and prepare for disasters in the following order:

1. Personal

2. Localized

3. Regional

4. State

5. National

6. Global

Losing a job, a family member, or experiencing a localized disaster, are the most likely threats you'll face. Plan and prepare for these first. Then, continue to address other concerns.

Most importantly, modern survivalism helps us build and design our lives. Jack Spirko puts it into perspective:

> "Your personal philosophy is more important for you than mine! You are the master of your own life and if you don't agree with my views, great – define, understand and implement your own. The biggest thing you can do is understand that you are in control of your life and that what you do matters. Those two factors have the greatest impact on individual survival across every demographic you can imagine."

Our lifestyle choices are so important! Choosing the modern survivalist lifestyle creates and (more importantly) maintains our overall health and well-being. That's why I'm a modern survivalist.

We can return to our roots by simplifying our lives, preparing for events that are very probable to happen in the future, forgetting about past events that only bring about stressful memories, and by talking to ourselves in a natural way. If we return to our roots, to who we truly are naturally, we will see a huge decrease in overall stress and a huge, overall increase in health and well-being.

We must realize that emotional symptoms like anxiety and depression are the consequence of a harmful amount of unnatural internal dialogue. We activate the stress response by not treating ourselves naturally and by talking to ourselves in an unnatural environment. The symptoms you experience when you do these things are just your mind telling you, "Something is wrong with my environment. Please change your internal dialogue." Depression is a symptom, not a cause. You feel depression, anxiety, and low self-esteem as emotional pain, just as you feel physical pain from cuts and bruises. Depression doesn't lead to depressing thoughts; depression is the consequence of depressing thoughts.

Depressing thoughts are harmful and destructive; happy thoughts on the other hand are natural and pure, and they build. With practice, you can become good at either choosing depressing thoughts or happy thoughts. Habits are created by repetitively stimulating neural pathways that form synapses; these habits can be healthy or not – that's your choice. Remember – this won't happen over night. You need to practice, work out, and maintain a training schedule just as you would have to in order to stay fit and healthy physically.

Movement
Not just for athletes!

I have two activities that I really enjoy, and I actually look for opportunities to do them. The first one is to work with a shovel and pick axe to move dirt, and the second is to chop wood with an axe. Most people right now are probably thinking, "this guy is weird." However, there are various reasons why I really enjoy these activities.

Well, first off, I guess you can say I am weird because I sincerely like digging in the dirt and chopping wood. Unfortunately, I don't get the opportunity to chop wood as much as I would like, however the last two times it was for an older lady who was living alone. My dad had bought some tree trunks that needed to be chopped, and I happily volunteered to help out by chopping all of it.

I also vividly remember this last summer being alone on my dad's land with a bottle of water and an axe, chopping wood. I was chopping the branches and trunk of a 60-year-old weeping willow that just the year before stood in the front yard of my parent's house. I remember many times sitting under this tree, enjoying the shade it left. It was the first tree I tried to build a tree house in when I was just a kid. This is the same tree that my brother fell from and broke his arm while we were trying to build that tree house.

Chopping the wood of this old willow tree, for example, are moments where I have the opportunity to really enjoy life and what surrounds me. I take the time to enjoy with each sense. I focus on the little things; feeling the grain of the wood I am lifting and placing on the block to chop next; touching and grabbing hold of the plastic handle of the axe; concentrating on not holding it too hard and focus on how it feels. Moments like these, I see the bugs flying around me, the different types of grass, the color of the flowers around me. I completely savor each drop of water that I drink, and as I work, I focus on the many different sounds around me. The different birds, bugs, wind ruffling between the leaves of the trees, and even the different sounds of vehicles on the I-15 highway not too far away. Also, I make sure each breath I take is deep, taking in the fresh clean air that surrounds me. How I love these opportunities to move and put weight against my muscles and bones.

You might not get any joy out of chopping wood, just like how I didn't find any joy in washing the dishes, until I starting doing the same thing I do when I chop wood. Focus your five senses on what you are doing. I focus on the texture of each dish I am washing, be it glass or plastic, round or flat. The sounds of the water, the soapy sponge gliding across a plate. The smell of the dirty and greasy dishes to those clean and recently rinsed. I see each part of each dish to make sure no grime is left behind and I remember how each food tasted. By focusing our five senses we can enjoy any activity, even those that are on the bottom of the list, but we must take the time and fully enjoy them.

For many, exercise would be one of the activities that they don't enjoy. No one can continually make the decision to do something they do not enjoy! It is against human nature. That is why so many people fail at their New Year's resolutions that have to do with weight loss or getting into shape. It is against human nature to continually do something that we perceive as not enjoyable. However, there is a way to change the belief system so many people have of exercise being painful and not enjoyable. If we truly focus our five senses when we do those supposedly not enjoyable activities we will find joy in them, and they become very easy to accomplish. Just like chopping wood brings me joy, running that extra mile or climbing that rope just one last time is not painful but truly enjoyable.

Recently my days have been very long, waking up early and going to bed late. These days also involve many hours of work in the sitting position. I recommend that you don't sit for more than 45 minutes at a time. I would get up and move a little before I went back at it, but over all, the day consisted of me sitting working in front of the computer. By the time it got into the afternoon, I was always tired and foggy.

Where we are living at the moment I am preparing the front yard to be able to plant vegetables. I am installing miniswales on contour. Swales are basically ditches that are level. What I want is the rain to fill them up evenly, not run off, and if they overflow to slowly go to the next miniswale letting the water slowly sink and spread into the soil below. Installing swales involves digging with a shovel, something I really enjoy. However, having been in the sitting position pretty much all day long, I was tired and felt foggy, and it was hard to find the will power to go out and dig in the soil. I found the fortitude and grabbed the shovel, went outside, and starting digging. I finished two miniswales and was able to finish the walking path between them by leveling it, placing cardboard down, and then pine wood chips on top of the cardboard. After doing that physically demanding work I was completely energized and felt great, not tired and foggy the way I felt just a couple of hours before. Movement wakes us up and energizes us! Sitting makes us tired and foggy!

Lack of movement has become a huge problem over the years. Modern society has made us into sedentary people. We are practically in the sitting position all day. We wake up to sit at a table, to then sit in a vehicle that takes us to our desk where we sit for another eight to nine hours. We then sit in our vehicle to go home to sit on the couch. Most people can relate to this in some way. Most movement is seen in either athletes or people that are either trying to lose weight or look better physically. However, that is where we have gone completely wrong.

Most people think that movement is something that is optional in our lifestyle, that it is not necessary to be healthy and well. Most people use exercise to either improve their sports performance, lose unwanted pounds, or to look better physically. As stated above, this is where we have gone completely wrong! Movement is so much more than that, it is a requirement for you to be truly healthy and well. We must move, and if you live a lifestyle where movement is not a common practice because of work or other responsibilities, you must plan time in your daily schedule for rigorous exercise. Lack of movement, a sedentary lifestyle, is harmful just like unnatural internal dialogue. In other words, it is a stressor. What happens when we stress the body? We activate the stress response, with all the stress hormones and other changes in our physiology that come with it.

We must remember that the activation of the stress response is a very intelligent thing our body does. If we are stressing our bodies in some way we need the stress response to survive; if we didn't have the stress response we would not survive the stressor. However, we are not designed to be stressed in a chronic fashion. If our bodies are chronically stressed, they become tired, fatigued, eventually sicken, and die.

Many professionals, when talking about the right amount of movement for our ecosystem of cells, recommend following the example of our Paleolithic ancestors. I continue to believe that we don't need to go back so far. Why go back 10,000 years when most of us only need to go back five or six generations to find in our own family line a more proper daily amount of exercise and movement?

There is a really neat documentary that I recommend called Polyfaces: A World of Many Choices. One of the people interviewed in this documentary was someone we could say had been living a normal modern life. He was sick and overweight and knew he needed a change. Throughout the film, this man progresses from being overweight and sick to the opposite; the change is quite dramatic and happens over time. What struck me was what this man said, and how the documentary portrayed his new lifestyle. He talked about how he had improved his lifestyle dramatically, which improved his overall health by leaps and bounds. He stated that what he did was begin to live a lifestyle like his grandparents. He was eating and moving the way he remembers his grandparents ate and moved. He was living a lifestyle of just two generations in the past. What I really like in the documentary is, after he explains his new lifestyle, it shows him chopping wood! What a great way to move!

The point I am trying to make is that if we go back just a couple generations we see a lifestyle of a lot more movement. This was natural to our ancestors. They woke up and moved. They didn't have gyms full of machines; they didn't have Zumba classes or any such thing. They lived a lifestyle that permitted them to move naturally. With today's technology we don't necessarily need to live how our ancestors lived, but we must emulate their lifestyle that involved a lot more movement.

Many of you reading this probably work behind a desk the majority of the day and are thinking how in the world am I supposed to move like my ancestors? That is why I say live their lifestyle of movement, not their way of life. However, if we are behind a desk the majority of the day and don't have many opportunities to move we must involve rigorous exercise to our lives.

I recommend exercising three to five days a week, and in most cases, five days a week is optimum. This exercise should last from thirty minutes to an hour and you should be breathing hard once you are done.

Of course if you are not accustomed to this type of movement you don't just start day one with an hour of highly intensive exercise. All these things come one step at a time. Many people will just start by walking, and that is great, but don't let that be the end goal. We must move more if we want to live a lifestyle of health and wellness.

The hard part is starting, but I can promise you that each and every one of us has the desire and the potential to start and stick to it. What I love about this lifestyle is that when you do start to move more you feel more energized and have the capacity to get a lot more accomplished throughout the day. It gets easier and easier with each day we involve more movement in our lives. We all can find time; when it comes to our health there is always time – we just need to be willing to make it important enough to always allow time to do it.

Sleep - movement's companion

I'm a person who really doesn't have too much of a problem with movement. Throughout my life, I have had great opportunities to stay active. I can't take the credit for staying active—it is thanks to many other people. For example, my parents have helped out. When I was young, they were so kind to let me help out in the garden. I had the great opportunity to weed a row a day, right after school. Who would have thought I would be thanking them now for that great opportunity!

I remember the majority of my childhood outside playing; sun or snow, it didn't matter. In the summer, my brothers and I would find huge piles of dirt and dig tunnels, making our very own ant hills. In winter, we would build walls and try to build igloos and have snowball wars. There was always an opportunity to move. As I grew, sports became a huge part of my life. I would play whenever I got the chance. I played all sorts of sports, from tackle football after school to basketball at five in the morning when my mom was doing aerobics (do you remember aerobics?) During high school, I played on the volleyball team, and I would also ride my bike to my aunt's house to swim on a hot day. I also became involved in new trends back in the day—skateboarding and snowboarding.

As life went on, I went through Marine Corps boot camp and continued to play sports and move in other ways, like hiking through the mountains with my family, or with my dad looking for that perfect elk. Today, I play basketball and soccer almost weekly while also walking and running to most places.

However, there is another part to movement, one most people would think has nothing to do with movement. They might also think it is unimportant. It is the opposite of movement. Sleep! Sleep has a very important part in our health and also with the assimilation of our movement during the day. Sleep is where I have had difficulties throughout certain periods of my life. I've had my share of internal struggles that kept me awake wondering "Can I?", "Am I capable?" or "Am I good enough?". Those have been hard times where my internal environment was not allowing me to fully assimilate the movement I was giving it. There have been many restless nights. Nights looking at the ceiling, opening up a book, twisting, turning, moving to the couch, returning to the bed and finally hearing the alarm clock one to two hours later. We need to view sleep as movement's companion. To fully take advantage of our movement, we must rest. But that is not all. We must rest for many more reasons as we move through this wonderful journey called wellness.

First off, how much sleep do we really need? That changes with age. For example, it's recommended that an infant should sleep between twelve and sixteen hours a day, including naps. Children between ages one and two should be sleeping between eleven and fourteen hours. Children aged between three and five are recommended to sleep ten to thirteen hours a day. Children between the ages of six and twelve are recommended to sleep nine to twelve hours. For teenagers, it is recommended they sleep between eight and ten hours a day. And for adults eighteen years and older, it is recommended they sleep between seven and eight hours a day. But it doesn't just have to do with hours of sleep; a lot has to do with quality of sleep. Many adults can get by with just six hours because they have learned how to achieve a very high quality of sleep.

The following table details the hours of sleep (including naps) recommended for each age group.

Age	Hours
Infants	12-16
1-2 years	11-14
3-5 years	10-13
6-12 years	9-12
Teenagers	8-10
Adults	7-8

If we ever want to reach our health potential we must rest. Sleeping—or in other words, recuperating—is incredibly important. Sleep effects us physically, mentally, and spiritually. Unfortunately, just like the food we eat, the way we talk to ourselves and the way we move, sleep has become completely unnatural. Most people think if you are getting enough sleep you are lazy. They think that they need less sleep to get more done. They couldn't be further from the truth. When we don't rest enough we become slower, less creative, and underperform. To truly be productive, we must rest.

With lights everywhere making the night seem like day, we think we can just stay awake until early in the morning. With the ability to light up the night, it might sound weird to most people that we should be going to sleep no more than a couple of hours after the sun goes down. It is said that the most productive hours of sleep are between ten p.m. and two a.m. That just makes sense, if we really think about it. Of course, this changes slightly depending on the season and the part of the world. As I always say, we are part of this ecosystem called Earth, not in control of it. As soon as we try to take control of nature using artificial light to stay up more hours, we are putting ourselves in a battle that we just can't win. And decreased health will be the consequence. Before artificial light, people went to bed when the sun went down. We should be doing the same!

One of the most important aspects of sleep is the cleaning out of the brain's metabolized waste byproducts. The brain works like any organ—it needs energy to work. Just like with movement, when we move, the energy used in an anaerobic manner, leaves us with heat and lactic acid. The lactic acid must be discarded or reused. As the brain uses energy, it leaves byproducts that must be discarded or reused. Normally, these wastes are discarded through the lymphatic system. However, our brain has a protective barrier called the blood brain barrier, where the lymphatic system does not pass. The brain has its own system to get rid of waste called the glymphatic system, the "g" added for the glial cells that control it. This system that rids the central nervous system of its byproducts is ten times more active when you are asleep than when you are awake. Not only that, but our brain cells actually reduce their size about sixty percent while we are asleep, making their job that much easier.

Not only is our brain cleaning up while we sleep, but it is preparing for the next day. While we are sleeping we are forming new neural pathways that help in the learning process and in our problem-solving skills. Getting a good night's rest also helps us pay attention, make better decisions, and be more creative.

Rest is also very important in our physical health, not just our mental health. As we sleep, we recuperate. Our immune system needs a good night's rest to be able to fight the good fight. Also, as we rest, we see an increase in growth hormone. This is where our muscle tissue grows. With rest we see an increase in the repair of damaged cells and tissues.

Other things we see with proper sleep are the adequate secretion of the "hungry" hormone, or ghrelin, and the "full" hormone, leptin. When we are sleep-deprived we see an increase in ghrelin and a decrease in leptin, causing us to be hungrier. We know the consequence of eating more of what society calls food, and we know it is not a good one. Another important part of sleep is the secretion of insulin. Just one night of not getting enough sleep can make us as insulin-resistant as a Type 2 diabetic. Sleep deprivation has huge affects on our health. Ongoing sleep deficiency has been linked to an increased risk of heart disease, kidney disease, high blood pressure, diabetes, and stroke.

Many people say they will take a nap during the day to recuperate the lost hours during the night. It just isn't the same! I am not saying naps are bad; they just can't replace a good night's rest. We have something called a circadian rhythm. We can call it our internal clock. Our bodies, being naturally intelligent, know when it is time to sleep. In other words, when the sun goes down there will be an increase in certain hormones that help us sleep, and when the sun comes up we will start to secrete different hormones to wake us and get us up and running. When we fail to do this we mess up this whole natural system, and over long periods of time, it will cause chaos in our health and well-being.

If we work with our natural internal clock—our circadian rhythm—and go to bed no more than a couple of hours after the sun goes down, we will have a natural and healthy secretion of a hormone called melatonin. This is the hormone most commonly known to help in the sleep-wake cycle. However, it has proved to be so much more. It is also a very potent antioxidant and probably one of the best anti-cancer hormones we produce. So not only does it help protect our cells and tissues, but it have been found to help protect us from cancer.

Other important hormones that naturally go up and down as the night turns to day, and the day turns to night, are serotonin and cortisol. I have already talked about these hormones, however they also have their roles in the sleep cycle. Serotonin—also known as the hormone that brings feelings of happiness—has a very important part in helping to regulate our internal clock. Not only is serotonin found in the digestive tract, it is also found in the skin, among other places. We have receptors in our eyes that send signals to our brains to increase the output of serotonin.

This serotonin can then be converted to melatonin. What I am really trying to get at is if we want a natural amount of serotonin that will then be converted to melatonin to help us get a good night's rest, we need to be outside moving in a natural manner, receiving the beautiful rays of the sun.

What about cortisol? Well, cortisol in our natural circadian system goes on an upswing when we are waking up. We secrete more cortisol in the morning to help us get up and to prepare us to take on the challenges of another day. It helps us stay awake and alert throughout the day. As the day goes on, the secretion continually goes down, finally bottoming out in the evening and setting us up to have a great night's sleep.

So it isn't just about sleeping more, but returning to who we truly are as human beings. We have the day to work hard, and we have the night to recuperate. If we truly want to be healthy—and I know you want to experience true health and well-being because you are reading this book—you need to return to living how humans have lived for thousands of years!

Moving is just half of the battle. If we want all the great effects of movement, we must rest. If we want a good night's rest, we must move. I am not talking about moving on the treadmill in some gym, with all sorts of artificial light. I am talking natural movement outside. We need to be receiving the sun's rays during the day, adequately moving as nature intended, so we can fully take advantage of the night hours to rest, repair, heal, and clean up.

Posture – the other side of the coin.

It is awkward to say this, but as I was writing this portion of the book I realized I was not sitting in the proper fashion and had to adjust my posture. Even the person behind all these pages is constantly reminding himself to maintain proper posture. Improper posture, the way we sit, the way we stand, has become just as epidemic as the sedentary lifestyle. We are not only sitting way too much, but we are sitting in a way that completely stresses the joints of our spine. We are completely deficient in movement and toxic in bad posture! We couldn't ask for a worse combination for the health of our spines and our overall health and well-being.

Someone recently asked me this question:

> "It is fairly obvious why exercise influences health. It is not as obvious (at least to me) why posture does. It seems to me that one's posture would have to deteriorate quite extensively before adversely affecting health, so I was wondering if you could describe in a bit more detail the mechanics associated with the process of bad posture leading to bad health?"

Exactly! It usually takes a long time for bad posture to actually cause a physical symptom like pain. Bad posture is one of the micro traumas that over time leads to so many health problems in our modern societies. I like to call the many metabolic diseases we see today as lifestyle diseases because they are completely preventable if we improve our current lifestyle to one that harmonizes with who we are naturally. Lifestyle diseases take decades to demonstrate. That's why I talk about the importance of wellness; this lifestyle prevents so much sickness and heartache. Bad posture has become a toxicity we put into our joints; it forces our bodies to adapt. When it becomes chronic, it causes many problems. Something we must recognize is that chronic not only means slow to demonstrate and have for prolonged periods of time, but it also means long to recuperate.

From the experience I have in clinic, people typically don't experience physical pain in their joints until later on in life, between the ages of thirty and sixty. Bad posture increases wear on our joints and causes an early onset of the inflammatory disease, osteoarthritis. It also decreases the overall number of nerve signals traveling between our brains and our extremities.

We now know that, besides osteoarthritis, our paleolithic ancestors did not suffer from the many metabolic diseases we suffer from today. I believe that the wear and tear of the joints of our paleolithic ancestors did not get to the point of causing physical symptoms besides short stiffness felt in the morning. Their joints wore out over time due to their daily activities. They had three of the pillars that allowed them live full, healthy and productive lives however they were lacking one vital pillar – chiropractic care! With chiropractic care they could have even prevented much of the degeneration of the joints of the spine.

For the last six years, posture has been a big part of my life. As a chiropractor, I focus on improving patients' postures. Chiropractic is important in regards to posture because the subluxation, the lesion I treat as a chiropractor, produces bad posture; on the other hand, bad posture is one cause of the subluxation. Since I started treating patients, I've focused on returning proper end range of motion to their joints so they can fully recuperate. End range of motion means the last few degrees of motion that patients often don't even notice they've lost. I also teach posture exercises to patients that give their soft tissue the strength to restore and maintain proper posture. This is one very important part to be able to return to true health and wellness.

Most of us in modern societies sit with poor postures for most of our lives. Unfortunately, this is beginning earlier and earlier in the developmental years where we are a lot more vulnerable to these unnatural postures.

Most people at least understand what a proper sitting posture looks like. However, try and maintain that position for more than a couple of minutes and let me know if it doesn't feel completely unnatural and uncomfortable. That's because of all the years of sitting in a completely unnatural posture. When you sit with proper posture, your joints and soft tissue feel stressed because they've adapted to your bad posture. In other words, your body is intelligent; it adapts to the best of its ability to the environments you put it in, including bad posture.

One example that I have a lot of experience in is the chronic anterior head carriage. This is when the opening of your ear canal is anterior from the center of your shoulder. What does this do to the normal cervical lordosis, also known as the normal curvature, or the reverse 'C' curve of the neck? Anterior head carriage or leaning your head forward decreases cervical lordosis. This puts gravitational forces forward onto the soft tissue in between the bones, which are called the intervertebral discs. This happens at the level of the fourth bone in the neck and below. Over time, this increased force leads to intervertebral disc degeneration and anterior osteophyte formation. In other words, an increase in the wear and tear of the tissues and bones that surround the joints.

However, with a normal cervical lordosis and normal head carriage, gravitational forces are equally placed between the two joints that are found at the back of each bone of the spine and the intervertebral disc; they each receive one-third of the weight. With anterior head carriage and the loss of the normal cervical lordotic curve, these forces are moved forward off of the two joints and onto the intervertebral disc and anterior portion of the vertebral body at the level of fourth neck bone and below.

This is why we see so much wear and tear on the anterior portion of the lower neck bones. The worst part about it is that it can take up to thirty years before there is enough scar tissue formed after this neural trauma to cause a physical symptom. This is occurring day after day, year after year, and we don't even know it is happening!

I this see quite often in clinical practice. Many patients in their 30's to early 60's make a primary complaint of constant neck pain or back pain for the first time; they often have no idea why they're experiencing pain. When I take radiographs, I almost always see the same thing: wear and tear at the front of the neck bones from the fourth neck bone down, and decreased space between the bones.

When I observe this condition, I examine patients' necks by touch and find their muscles are tense and tender to the touch. Even when patients come in with no neck pain, I can find areas of discomfort and tense muscles by examining their necks.

This is due to the years of chronic sitting and anterior head carriage. In other words, this is caused by bad posture at desks in front of computers, on couches in front of televisions, when using electronic devices like iPads or iPhones, and driving, just to name a few. The worst part is, this condition is happening earlier and earlier in modern societies. It's impossible to put the human spine through the following chronic stressors without harmful effects: sitting, traumas (especially micro traumas), sedentary lifestyles, poor nutrition, and increased emotional stress. These are the reasons why pretty much everybody in modern societies suffers from subluxation and bad posture.

Bad posture not only effects the joints and soft tissue around them over time. Bad posture affects almost all human functions, both conscious and unconscious, from movement to breathing. This is realized by the increase in the nociceptive input and the decrease in the proprioceptive input of the stressed joint that I have already talked about.

Most people understand the importance of going to a dentist regularly. We brush and floss our teeth to prevent cavities, we understand that our modern diet has way too many carbohydrates, which are just long chains of sugars and too much refined sugars that causes tooth decay. In the same way, modern activity patterns and the unnatural postural patterns we see in modern society have caused spinal decay, very little movement, and low overall health levels. Modern living leads to the subluxation and subsequent wear and tear in our joints. Receiving chiropractic care on a regular basis balances the effects of modern activity patterns that result in bad posture. Chiropractic care is as crucial for spinal health as dental care is for healthy teeth!

Movement and posture go hand in hand and are vital pillars in our health and well-being. As we return to who we are naturally and begin to move more and more, and use proper posture, the system of belief that movement is not enjoyable will fade away and we will truly be on the path to increased health, energy, vitality, and will return to how we as humans should look and feel. We need to remember that we cannot replace one for the other. We cannot go to a chiropractor thinking that the movement he returns to our joints and improved posture is enough, and we cannot think that just more movement on our own part is enough. Spinal health and proper posture are needed so the movement that we provide that is so vital to our health can reach our brain and be fully processed.

Why We Must Get the Word Out!

I was covering for a chiropractor in Las Vegas, NV during the time he was on vacation. I saw quite a few patients during the four days I was at that clinic. I saw again firsthand what's wrong with the American health paradigm, and unfortunately it is spreading all over the world. We have to get the word out about the wellness paradigm.

This won't be an easy task. It's as if a huge cargo ship has left port and traveled a long distance. Suddenly, the captain realizes a huge storm is coming and has to turn the ship around and head back. Modern medicine is this huge cargo ship; it can't just stop and make a 180-degree turn. It takes a lot of energy to turn around a ship of that size. However, if we don't turn our ship around, we'll head right into a huge storm, and we'll be shipwrecked. We need to start making changes now, one degree at a time. If we stay constant, we'll get this huge ship turned around and facilitate a much-needed change in world health. To turn this ship around one degree at a time, each of us must learn and implement the four pillars of health and wellness in our lives. Then, one-by-one, we can help our families and communities understand and implement these principles in their lives.

We need to return to how human beings once lived. There's nothing new to what I'm teaching. We need to return to eating local food that is in season that is grown or raised on soil that is alive without chemicals. We need to return to planting some of our own food. Everybody needs to know how to save seed, build soil, and grow food, from the farmer with thousands of acres, to the city dweller with only a balcony. Everybody can grow a percentage of their own food even if it's just 1 percent of their total consumption.

The main reason why we must all be growing some of our own food is because it is the freshest and most nutritious food you and your family can get. Get everything else from the most local possible sources. Befriend your local farmers; make sure they're growing vegetables without chemicals in living soil. If you know your local farmers, you can be sure you're consuming properly raised meats. Animals should be outside with the sun on their backs and the grass under their feet!

We must eat more properly raised vegetables and meats that have the nutrients our bodies require. We need to accompany these vegetables and meats with fruits and small portions of carbohydrates. Of course, we need to completely eliminate processed foods from our diets; our foods shouldn't need labels. You might say that sounds ridiculous, but just over seventy years ago, that's how it was. Before the first supermarkets cropped up in America in the 1940's, our food came from homes, gardens, local farms, and forests.

We can return to that way of life! We can return, but with new abilities. Just imagine what we can do with today's technology and yesterday's knowledge. The possibilities are enormous.

We need to return to thinking naturally. We need to realize human beings are born with certain natural values; the basis of all of them is unconditional love. If we base all of our belief systems on our natural values, we human beings will think naturally and use natural internal dialogues. This change will bring about natural interactions with each other. As Melvin Konner, M.D., Ph.D. author of The Paleolithic Prescription(1) wrote:

> "Imagine an infancy in which your needs for love and physical closeness were indulged, a childhood that - if you escaped serious illness - allowed you to flourish and mature at your own rate, absorbing and learning from role models only slightly older than yourself, a reasonably carefree adolescence that promoted individualism and self-confidence, assured you of your physical attractiveness and didn't expect you to assume full adult responsibilities until you reached your late teens...Imagine, as well, an adulthood that essentially guaranteed marriage (with room for divorce and remarriage if necessary),

that made it likely that you would have children, yet would not ostracize you if you couldn't or isolate you if you did, and that had social supports enabling you to balance family obligations with significant contributions to the economy. Although age, accidents, and infectious disease would gradually decrease your physical capabilities, your status within the community, especially within your family group, would be likely to increase. You would be turned to for the knowledge you possess about the past, highly relevant to a world that changes slowly, if at all."

We can return to this natural way of life and live meaningful lives, not only for ourselves, but those around us. We can use natural internal dialogue, like our ancestors. We can align our belief systems with our natural values.

We need to return to getting proper and natural movement every day, not to improve sports performance, lose weight, or look better, but because it's vital to our health. We as human beings are naturally and genetically made to move.

A lot of our movement should be in nature. Our feet need to touch the living soil; we need to touch trees and plants as we move. We need to feel, see, hear, smell and taste what surrounds us. We need to more fully enjoy movement!

If you can't move more due to your circumstances, you must move with more intensity. You don't have to move all day; you just need to move with more intensity and eat a diet of whole foods. Don't forget this vital pillar in your health and well-being; if you neglect or forget to move, you're moving backward toward sickness – not forward toward wellness and health.

It was stated beautifully in the medical article, "Waging war on physical inactivity: using modern molecular ammunition against an ancient enemy"(2):

> "Physical inactivity is an abnormal event for genes that are programmed to expect physical activity. This helps explain, in part, how physical inactivity leads to metabolic dysfunctions and eventual metabolic disorders such as atherosclerosis, hypertension, obesity, type 2 diabetes, and so forth...It is likely that humans have an intrinsic biological requirement for a certain threshold of physical activity, with a sedentary lifestyle being a disruption of the normal homeostatic mechanisms programmed for proper metabolic flux needed to maintain health."

We must maintain proper end range of motion in our joints to prevent wear and tear. We also must receive chiropractic care to prevent the degradation of our spinal joints. These joints make up one of the four walls from which each nerve root that branches off of the spinal cord passes through. These nerves innervate our entire bodies. They innervate the muscles we use for mobility and to move blood through our arteries; they innervate all of our organs, from our livers to our reproductive organs. Our nervous system is the most neglected organ in our bodies.

We use chiropractic care to prevent many conditions. It reduces the negative health effects of nociception and increases the proprioception our central nervous system receives. The more proprioception that gets to our central nervous systems, the less nociception we experience. Nociception includes stressful and noxious stimuli from our environments: physical stressors like subluxation (the lesion I treat as a chiropractor), toxic stressors like the processed foods we ingest, mental stressors, and our negative internal dialogues.

We can change the course of our huge cargo ship headed straight into the storm of poor health. We can do this one degree at a time – one person at a time. We can accomplish this by understanding and implementing the four pillars of health and wellness in our lives. By holistically combining nutrient dense food that is grown on soil that is alive without chemicals, adequate movement, natural internal dialogue, and chiropractic care, we can achieve true health and wellness.

Let's get out there and live our lives just a little bit better – one day at a time!

[1] Eaton B, Shostak M, and Konner, M. The Paleolithic Prescription. Harper and Row; 1988

[2] Booth, et al. Waging war on physical inactivity: using modern molecular ammunition against an ancient enemy. J appl physiol. 2002; 93: 3-30

Printed in Great Britain
by Amazon